The AOTA Practice Guidelines Series

Occupational Therapy Practice Guidelines *for* Adults With Stroke

Joyce S. Sabari, PhD, OTR, FAOTA
Associate Professor and Chairperson
Occupational Therapy Program
State University of New York
Downstate Medical Center
Brooklyn

Deborah Lieberman, MHSA, OTR/L, FAOTA
Series Editor
Program Director, Evidence-Based Practice
Staff Liaison to the Commission on Practice
American Occupational Therapy Association
Bethesda, MD

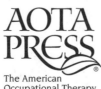

AOTA PRESS
The American Occupational Therapy Association, Inc.

Centennial Vision

We envision that occupational therapy is a powerful, widely recognized, science-driven, and evidence-based profession with a globally connected and diverse workforce meeting society's occupational needs.

Vision Statement

The American Occupational Therapy Association advances occupational therapy as the pre-eminent profession in promoting the health, productivity, and quality of life of individuals and society through the therapeutic application of occupation.

Mission Statement

The American Occupational Therapy Association advances the quality, availability, use, and support of occupational therapy through standard-setting, advocacy, education, and research on behalf of its members and the public.

AOTA Staff

Frederick P. Somers, *Executive Director*
Christopher M. Bluhm, *Chief Operating Officer*

Chris Davis, *Director, AOTA Press*
Michael N. Melletz, *Book and Journal Production Manager*
Ashley Hofmann, *Production Editor*
Victoria Davis, *Editorial Assistant*

Beth Ledford, *Director, Marketing and Member Communications*

The American Occupational Therapy Association, Inc.
4720 Montgomery Lane
Bethesda, MD 20814
Phone: 301-652-AOTA (2682)
TDD: 800-377-8555
Fax: 301-652-7711
www.aota.org
To order: 1-877-404-AOTA (2682)

Disclaimers

This publication is designed to provide accurate and authoritative information in regard to the subject matter covered. It is sold or distributed with the understanding that the publisher is not engaged in rendering legal, accounting, or other professional services. If legal advice or other expert assistance is required, the services of a competent professional person should be sought.
—*From the Declaration of Principles jointly adopted by the American Bar Association and a*
   Committee of Publishers and Associations

It is the objective of the American Occupational Therapy Association to be a forum for free expression and interchange of ideas. The opinions expressed by the contributors to this work are their own and not necessarily those of the American Occupational Therapy Association.

ISBN-13: 978-1-56900-263-6

Library of Congress Control Number: 2008937072

Design by Sarah Ely and Michael N. Melletz
Printed by Automated Graphic Systems, Inc., White Plains, MD.

Contents

References 145

Tables, Figures, and Boxes Used in This Publication

Acknowledgments

The author would like to acknowledge the following individuals for their contributions to the evidence-based literature review:

Marian Arbesman, PhD, OTR/L
Catherine Trombly Latham, ScD, OTR/L, FAOTA
Hui-ing Ma, ScD, OTR

The author also thanks the following individuals for their participation in the content review and development of this publication:

Marian Arbesman, PhD, OTR/L
Susan Fasoli, ScD, OTR/L
Nancy Flinn, PhD, OTR/L

Glen Gillen, EdD, OTR, FAOTA
Margo Johnson, MA
Catherine Trombly Latham, ScD, OTR/L, FAOTA
Kathryn Levit, PhD, OTR/L
Judy Thomas, MGA
Anne Woodson, OTR

The author thanks the following individuals for their participation in the development of the case studies included in this publication:

Claribell Bayonna, BS, OTR/L
Rachel Feld-Glazman, MS, OTR/L
Robin Silver, OTR/L

Introduction

Purpose and Use of This Publication

Practice guidelines have been widely developed in response to the health care reform movement in the United States. Such guidelines can be a useful tool for improving the quality of health care, enhancing consumer satisfaction, promoting appropriate use of services, and reducing costs. The American Occupational Therapy Association (AOTA), which represents 38,000 occupational therapists, occupational therapy assistants, and students of occupational therapy, is committed to providing information to support decision making that promotes a high-quality health care system that is affordable and accessible to all.

Using an evidence-based perspective and key concepts from the *Occupational Therapy Practice Framework: Domain and Process* (AOTA, 2008b), this Guideline provides an overview of the occupational therapy process for stroke. It defines the occupational therapy domain, process, and intervention that occurs within the boundaries of acceptable practice. This Guideline does not discuss all possible methods of care. Although it does recommend some specific methods of care, the occupational therapist makes the ultimate judgment regarding the appropriateness of a given procedure in light of a specific person's circumstances and needs.

Through this publication, it is the intent of AOTA to help occupational therapists and occupational therapy assistants, as well as those who manage, reimburse, or set policy regarding occupational therapy services, understand the contribution of occupational therapy in treating adults with stroke. This Guideline also can serve as a reference for other health care professionals, health care facility managers, education and health care regulators, third-party payers, and managed care organizations. This document may be used in any of the following ways:

- To assist occupational therapists and occupational therapy assistants in communicating about their services to external audiences
- To assist other health care practitioners and program administrators in determining whether referral for occupational therapy services would be appropriate
- To assist third-party payers in determining the medical necessity for occupational therapy
- To assist health and education planning teams in determining the need for occupational therapy
- To assist legislators, third-party payers, and administrators in understanding the professional education, training, and skills of occupational therapists and occupational therapy assistants
- To assist program developers, administrators, legislators, and third-party payers in understanding the scope of occupational therapy services
- To assist program evaluators and policy analysts in this practice area in determining outcome measures for analyzing the effectiveness of occupational therapy intervention
- To assist policy, education, and health care benefit analysts in understanding the appropriateness of occupational therapy services for stroke
- To assist occupational therapy educators in designing appropriate curricula that prepare future occupational therapy practitioners to work with adults with stroke.

The introduction to this Guideline continues with a brief discussion of the domain and process of occupational therapy. This discussion is followed by a detailed description of the occupational therapy process for stroke survivors and evidence-based practice as it relates to occupational therapy, including a summary of evidence from the literature regarding best practices with people who have experienced a stroke. Finally, the appendixes contain additional information about occupational therapists and occupational therapy assistants, the evidence-based literature review, and other resources related to occupational therapy for stroke survivors.

Domain and Process of Occupational Therapy

A hallmark of occupational therapy is its knowledge of occupation and of how engaging in occupations can be used to improve human performance and ameliorate the effects of disease and disability (AOTA, 2008b).

In 2002, the AOTA Representative Assembly adopted the *Occupational Therapy Practice Framework: Domain and Process.* Informed by the previous *Uniform Terminology for Occupational Therapy* (AOTA, 1979, 1989, 1994) and the World Health Organization's (2001) *International Classification of Functioning, Disability, and Health,* the *Framework* outlines the profession's domain and the process of service delivery within this domain. The second edition of the *Occupational Therapy Practice Framework* was published in 2008.

Domain

A profession's domain articulates its sphere of knowledge, societal contribution, and intellectual or scientific activity. The occupational therapy profession's domain centers on helping others participate in daily life activities. The broad term that the profession uses to describe daily life activities is *occupation.* As outlined in the *Framework,* occupational therapists and occupational therapy assistants[1] work collaboratively with clients to support participation through engagement in occupation (see Figure 1). This overarching mission circumscribes the profession's domain and emphasizes the important ways in which environmental and life circumstances influence the manner in which people

carry out their occupations. Key terms of the domain of occupational therapy are defined in Box 1.

Process

Many professions use the process of evaluating, intervening, and targeting outcomes that is outlined in the *Framework.* Occupational therapy's application of this process is made unique, however, by its focus on occupation (see Figure 2). The process of occupational therapy service delivery begins with the occupational profile, an assessment of the client's occupational needs, problems, and concerns; and the analysis of occupational performance, which includes the performance skills, performance patterns, contexts, activity demands, and client factors that contribute to or impede the client's satisfaction with his or her ability to engage in valued daily life activities. Therapists then plan and implement intervention using a variety of approaches and methods in which occupation is both the means and the end goal (Trombly, 1995). Occupational therapists continually assess the effectiveness of the intervention and the client's progress toward targeted outcomes. The intervention review informs decisions to continue or discontinue intervention and to make referrals to other agencies or professionals. Therapists select outcome measures that are valid, reliable, and appropriately sensitive to the client's occupational performance, satisfaction, adaptation, role competence, health and wellness, and quality of life.

Occupational therapy outcome goals may be *restorative* or *compensatory.* Restorative intervention seeks to change factors within a person that affect performance in areas of occupation. Intervention focuses on attaining restorative goals when the person shows potential and desire for change in body functions, performance skills, or patterns of performance. Restorative intervention includes the use of selected therapeutic procedures designed to promote recovery or change

---

[1] *Occupational therapists* are responsible for all aspects of occupational therapy service delivery and are accountable for the safety and effectiveness of the occupational therapy service delivery process. *Occupational therapy assistants* deliver occupational therapy services under the supervision of and in partnership with occupational therapists (AOTA, 2004). When the term *occupational therapy practitioner* is used in this document, it refers to both occupational therapists and occupational therapy assistants (AOTA, 2006).

Areas of Occupation	Client Factors	Performance Skills	Performance Patterns	Context and Environment	Activity Demands
Activities of daily living (ADLs)*	Values, beliefs, and spirituality	Sensory perceptual skills	Habits	Cultural	Objects used and their properties
Instrumental activities of daily living (IADLs)	Body functions	Motor and praxis skills	Routines	Personal	Space demands
Rest and sleep	Body structures	Emotional regulation skills	Roles	Physical	Social demands
Education		Cognitive skills	Rituals	Social	Sequencing and timing
Work		Communication and social skills		Temporal	Required actions
Play				Virtual	Required body functions
Leisure					Required body structures
Social participation					
*Also referred to as *basic activities of daily living (BADLs)* or *personal activities of daily living (PADLs)*.					

Figure 1. Aspects of occupational therapy's domain.
All aspects of the domain transact to support engagement, participation, and health. This figure does not imply a hierarchy.

Note. From *Occupational Therapy Practice Framework: Domain and Process, 2nd Edition,* by American Occupational Therapy Association, 2008, *American Journal of Occupational Therapy, 62,* pp. 628–645. Copyright © 2008 by American Occupational Therapy Association. Reprinted with permission.

Evaluation

Occupational profile—The initial step in the evaluation process that provides an understanding of the client's occupational history and experiences, patterns of daily living, interests, values, and needs. The client's problems and concerns about performing occupations and daily life activities are identified, and the client's priorities are determined.

Analysis of occupational performance—The step in the evaluation process during which the client's assets, problems, or potential problems are more specifically identified. Actual performance is often observed in context to identify what supports performance and what hinders performance. Performance skills, performance patterns, context or contexts, activity demands, and client factors are all considered, but only selected aspects may be specifically assessed. Targeted outcomes are identified.

Intervention

Intervention plan—A plan that will guide actions taken and that is developed in collaboration with the client. It is based on selected theories, frames of reference, and evidence. Outcomes to be targeted are confirmed.

Intervention implementation—Ongoing actions taken to influence and support improved client performance. Interventions are directed at identified outcomes. Client's response is monitored and documented.

Intervention review—A review of the implementation plan and process as well as its progress toward targeted outcomes.

Outcomes *(Supporting Health and Participation in Life Through Engagement in Occupation)*

Outcomes—Determination of success in reaching desired targeted outcomes. Outcome assessment information is used to plan future actions with the client and to evaluate the service program (i.e., program evaluation).

Figure 2. Process of occupational therapy service delivery.
The process of service delivery is applied within the profession's domain to support the client's health and participation.

Note. From *Occupational Therapy Practice Framework: Domain and Process, 2nd Edition,* by American Occupational Therapy Association, 2008. *American Journal of Occupational Therapy, 62,* p. 646. Copyright © 2008, American Occupational Therapy Association. Reprinted with permission.

Box 1. Key Terms From the *Framework*

Performance in areas of occupation:

The broad range of life activities in which people engage, including
- Activities of daily living that are oriented to taking care of one's own body, such as bathing (Rogers & Holm, 1994)
- Instrumental activities that are oriented toward interacting with the environment, such as home management (Rogers & Holm, 1994)
- Rest and sleep activities related to obtaining restorative rest and sleep that supports healthy active engagement in other areas of occupation
- Education that incorporates activities needed for being a student and participating in a learning environment
- Work activities needed for engaging in remunerative employment or volunteer activities (Mosey, 1996, p. 341)
- Play activities that provide enjoyment, amusement, or diversion (Parham & Fazio, 1997, p. 252)
- Leisure activities that people engage in during discretionary time (Parham & Fazio, 1997, p. 250)
- Social participation activities that involve interactions with community, family, and friends (Mosey, 1996, p. 340).

Performance skills:

Abilities clients demonstrate in the actions they perform. Includes sensory–perceptual, motor and praxis, emotional regulation, cognitive, and communication and social skills.

Performance patterns:

Established modes of behavior related to habits, routines, rituals, and roles.

Contexts and environments:

The array of interrelated conditions within and surrounding an individual that influence performance, including cultural, personal, temporal, virtual, physical, and social.

Activity demands:

The aspects of an activity, including the objects and their physical properties, space, social demands, sequencing or timing, required actions or skills, and required underlying body functions and body structure needed to carry out the activity (AOTA, 2008b).

Client factors:

Those factors residing within the client and that may affect performance in areas of occupation (AOTA, 2008b), including values, beliefs and spirituality, body functions, and body structures.

Note. Adapted from *Occupational Therapy Practice Framework: Domain and Process, 2nd Edition,* by American Occupational Therapy Association, 2008, *American Journal of Occupational Therapy, 62,* pp. 631–638. Copyright © 2008 by American Occupational Therapy Association. Adapted with permission.

in body functions, such as muscle strength or cognitive ability. Restorative intervention also includes therapeutic practice to improve performance skills and performance patterns. Compensatory interventions include adaptations to activity demands and the performance context that enable a person to resume performance of valued occupations, even when deficits in body functions, performance skills, or performance patterns are not amenable to change.

Occupational Therapy Process for Stroke Survivors

Of the 700,000 people in the United States who experience a new or recurrent stroke each year, more than 500,000 survive. More than 1.1 million adults in the United States report difficulties related to functional limitations resulting from stroke (American Heart Association/American Stroke Association, 2007). Depending on the site and the extent of neural damage, stroke survivors must cope with varying degrees of residual impairments. Common stroke sequelae include hemiplegia or hemiparesis, balance deficits, aphasia, cognitive deficits, sensory loss, and disorders in sensory processing (Jorgensen et al., 1995). Poststroke fatigue is an additional impairment, experienced by at least half of all stroke survivors (Choi-Kwon, Han, Kwon, & Kim, 2005; Ingles, Eskes, & Phillips, 1999). These deficits dramatically affect a person's ability to perform valued occupations safely and independently (Fong, Chan, & Au, 2001). Some 50–70% of stroke survivors regain functional independence, but 15–30% are permanently disabled. Twenty percent require institutional care at 3 months after onset (American Heart Association/American Stroke Association, 2007).

The focus of medical intervention after stroke is to limit the physiological impact of the stroke and, thus, the extent of residual impairments. In addition, medical or surgical procedures are instituted to prevent a recurrent stroke. Because damaged cells in the human central nervous system do not regenerate, stroke survivors cannot implicitly expect recovery with time and rest. Fortunately, however, there is evidence that the remaining healthy neural structures have the capacity to reorganize with subsequent improvements in behavioral function. Current research with primates and humans (Dahlqvist, Ronnback, Bergstrom, Soderstrom, & Olsson, 2004; Schaechter, 2004) indicates that this plasticity is influenced by environmental challenges in the form of activity demands. Unfortunately, environmental challenges also may foster the development of secondary impairments that seriously limit the abilities of stroke survivors to use reemerging motor or cognitive skills. Secondary impairments are preventable deficits that develop over time in response to immobility, inactivity, or asymmetries in postural alignment. Loss of muscle length, limitations in joint range of motion, diminished flexibility between body segments, pain, and edema are common secondary impairments in stroke survivors. Psychological depression and learned nonuse of a paretic arm may also be viewed as preventable, secondary impairments.

Occupational therapy practitioners are critical rehabilitation professionals for stroke survivors. Through prevention of secondary impairments and provision of individually selected environmental challenges, occupational therapists and occupational therapy assistants maximize functional recovery and enable people to apply reemerging skills in their functional performance of daily tasks. In addition, occupational therapy practitioners enable people to continue their participation in valued activities, even with remaining motor, cognitive, and perceptual impairments. A comprehensive occupational therapy program for any stroke survivor will artfully target both restorative and compensatory outcome goals. Improvements in motor, cognitive, perceptual, and other skills alone, unaccompanied by adaptations to activity demands or physical accessibility, may fail to lead to an outcome of full, meaningful participation. Correspondingly, overreliance on compensation without providing opportunities to improve performance skills seriously limits stroke survivors from reaching their ultimate potential for engagement in a wide variety of life roles.

Stages of Intervention

Occupational therapy practitioners may provide intervention to stroke survivors with a wide range of neurological impairments in a variety of settings and at various lengths of time after the acute stroke. This document refers to three stages of stroke recovery:
- The acute stage immediately following stroke
- The rehabilitation stage
- The stage of continuing adjustment.

Occupational therapy evaluation and intervention will vary on the basis of a person's stage and pattern of stroke recovery, the intervention setting, the environment in which the stroke survivor resides, and the extent of impairment. In addition, each person's individual goals and interests will significantly influence the occupational therapy process.

For the purposes of this Guideline, the *acute stage* is the initial days following the stroke. Stroke survivors at the acute stage are hospital inpatients, either in the intensive care unit, a designated stroke unit, or a neurological unit. The focus of occupational therapy intervention is on preventing the development of secondary impairments and maximizing recovery of motor and cognitive function.

Some stroke survivors at the *rehabilitation stage* reside temporarily at a rehabilitation facility or a subacute facility, where they participate in an integrated program of rehabilitation therapies. Others return to their homes and participate in home-based or outpatient rehabilitation. The goals initiated during the acute stage—to prevent development of secondary impairments and to maximize recovery—continue during rehabilitation. However, two important new focuses are added: Occupational therapy intervention promotes skills and activity patterns within the parameters of reemerging motor and cognitive function and also promotes safe and independent occupational performance within the parameters and constraints of available recovery.

The *stage of continuing adjustment* begins with discharge from a rehabilitation program. Stroke survivors who can function safely in their own homes face daily challenges in structuring their activities and routines to adapt to their current skills. Stroke survivors with more limited recovery or family resources are discharged to long-term nursing homes or assisted living settings where they strive to maintain independent activity performance and meaningful role engagement within a supported environment.

Referral

Referrals for occupational therapy stroke services during the acute stage are generated by attending physicians or other medical professionals as soon as the diagnosis of stroke is established and life-threatening problems are under control (Duncan et al., 2005). Services often begin within the first 24 hours after a stroke (Langhorne & Pollock, 2002). Referrals may request initial screening for cognitive deficits. Results of cognitive screening determine the need for cognitive reorientation and may influence discharge decisions in later stages of recovery. At many facilities, occupational therapists routinely assess swallowing skills to determine the need for dysphagia interventions. Patients with significant paralysis are referred to occupational therapy for positioning and improving passive range of motion to prevent development of secondary motor impairments. Patients with higher levels of cognitive and motor function may be referred to occupational therapy to begin immediate intervention for restoration of performance skills to prestroke levels.

Referrals during the rehabilitation stage are typically generated by a psychiatrist or other medical professional who requests a comprehensive evaluation (assessment) and intervention to maximize the person's potential for recovery and participation in daily activities. Occupational therapy is an integral component of the interdisciplinary services provided to stroke survivors in rehabilitation facilities, subacute rehabilitation facilities, home health programs, and outpatient programs.

Many stroke survivors and their families require occupational therapy intervention at different times after the formal stage of rehabilitation. Whenever a stroke survivor changes his or her living environment, occupational therapy referral may be indicated to assess the environmental impact on occupational (activity) performance and to implement changes in equipment, strategies, or home design that will maximize safety and independence in valued activities. Referrals for stroke survivors who reside in long-term-care facilities may specifically request occupational therapy assessment and intervention to improve posture and enhance physical comfort through appropriate bed and wheelchair positioning.

Stroke survivors who resume participation in their prestroke communities may request referral to intermittent occupational therapy services for a variety of reasons. The person may need to develop skills and abilities in performing new activities because of changes in his or her context. Examples include learning to drive an automobile; learning child care or homemaking skills; learning to maneuver in a newly purchased car or van; accessing technology for communication, computer use, or mobility; and learning to perform daily tasks in a new environment. In addition, the person may show evidence of improved motor functioning and be a candidate for learning to perform daily activities while standing or walking, or learning to incorporate the paretic upper extremity into task performance. Furthermore, cognitive or perceptual deficits that were previously undetected may be revealed through comprehensive evaluations for driving or return to work, and the person may become a candidate for a cognitive or perceptual retraining program.

Access to short-term occupational therapy services at critical points during the ongoing adjustment stage after stroke may influence quality of life, safety, and capacity to continue independent living (Logan et al., 2004; Widen-Holmqvist et al., 1993).

Evaluation

Occupational therapists perform evaluations in collaboration with clients and target information specific to the desired outcomes. The two elements of the occupational therapy evaluation are the *occupational profile* and the *analysis of occupational performance* (AOTA, 2008b).

Occupational Profile

The purpose of the occupational profile is to determine potential goals on the basis of the person's recent roles—in family relationships, social networks, work, and leisure pursuits. Through interview or formal assessment, the occupational therapist determines the person's concerns with regard to meeting task demands in daily life. Formal assessments may include the Canadian Occupational Performance Measure (COPM; Law et al., 1998) and time configuration evaluations, in which the client reflects on a typical day and records in half-hour increments how he or she spends time. The Motor Activity Log (MAL; van der Lee, Beckerman, Knol, de Vet, & Bouter, 2004) is an assessment that, although usually viewed as a measure of performance skills (i.e., skilled arm and hand function), can provide an additional dimension to information gathered through the occupational profile. This tool asks stroke survivors to rate the amount and the effectiveness of use of their paretic upper limb during selected daily tasks. It can serve as a valuable guide for the occupational therapist in determining which aspects of arm function are most important to specifically assess before planning treatment goals and interventions.

In developing the occupational profile, the therapist
- Determines why the client is seeking services
- Identifies the areas of occupation in which the client is successful and those in which the client has problems
- Identifies the contexts and environments that support and inhibit engagement in occupations
- Discusses significant aspects of the client's occupational history
- Determines the client's priorities and desired outcomes.

During the acute stage after stroke, the occupational profile is secondary to an assessment of client factors and performance skills. During the stages of rehabilitation and continuing adjustment, however, occupational therapists must understand the needs and expectations of the client and family in order to assess pertinent aspects of occupational performance, establish targeted outcomes collaboratively, and plan intervention.

Analysis of Occupational Performance

The occupational therapist uses information from the occupational profile to focus on the specific areas of occupation within the client's current context. When analyzing occupational performance the therapist

- *Observes the client* as he or she performs the occupations in the natural or least restrictive environment and notes the effectiveness of the client's performance skills and performance patterns
- *Selects specific assessments and assessment methods* that will identify and measure the factors that may be influencing the client's performance (see Table 1 for examples of selected assessments)
- *Interprets the assessment data* to identify what supports or hinders performance
- *Develops or refines a hypothesis* regarding the client's performance
- *Develops goals in collaboration with the client* that address the client's desired outcomes
- *Identifies potential intervention approaches,* guided by best practice and the evidence, and discusses them with the client
- *Documents the evaluation process and communicates the results* to the appropriate team members and community agencies.

Areas of Occupation

On the basis of the client's age and current lifestyle, the occupational therapist assesses his or her ability to perform basic and instrumental activities of daily living, rest and sleep activities, work activities, leisure activities, activities related to family roles (e.g., parent, grandparent), and activities related to participation in community and social pursuits.

Performance Skills

Stroke survivors present with skill deficits in arm and hand function, balance, functional ambulation, cognition, perception, and communication that range in type and severity. The purpose of assessing performance skills is to determine the extent to which a stroke survivor is able to actively use the motor and cognitive abilities that either have been spared by or recovered after the stroke. Occupational therapists are qualified to administer both standardized and observational assessments of performance skills.

Client Factors

Client factors are the underlying abilities that allow for skilled performance. The client factors of interest in stroke survivors are the primary and secondary impairments associated with stroke. Common primary impairments of interest to occupational therapy practitioners are motor paralysis, sensory loss, and cognitive and perceptual deficits. The occupational therapist must assess these factors to determine current potential for improvements in skills and occupational performance. Secondary impairments are the preventable client factors that, if allowed to develop, will present further obstacles to skill development and performance of valued activities. The occupational therapist assesses joint range of motion, postural alignment, fatigue, limb edema, skin integrity, and emotional adjustment to identify early problems and implement treatment to prevent further decline. Most of these assessment procedures require specific training, which is a core component of occupational therapy education. In addition, many stroke survivors have other significant comorbid health conditions that the occupational therapist must consider when developing the plan of care.

Performance Patterns

The habits, routines, roles, and rituals of a person's daily life (*performance patterns*) contribute significantly

Table 1. Selected Assessments Used by Occupational Therapists With Stroke Survivors

Aspects of the Domain of Occupational Therapy	Specific Functions Within Each Aspect	Examples of Specific Assessments Used in Occupational Therapy Practice
Areas of Occupation	■ Activities of daily living ■ Instrumental activities of daily living ■ Rest and sleep ■ Education ■ Work ■ Leisure ■ Social participation	■ Canadian Occupational Performance Measure (COPM; Law et al., 1998) ■ Stroke Impact Scale (Duncan et al., 1999; Duncan, Bode, Min Lai, & Perera, 2003) ■ Functional Independence Measure (Center for Functional Assessment Research, 1993) ■ Kohlman Evaluation of Living Skills (Thomson, 1992) ■ Assessment of Motor and Process Skills (AMPS; Fischer, 1995) ■ Role checklist (Oakley, Kielhofner, Barris, & Reichler, 1986) ■ Self-assessment of Leisure Interests (Kautzmann, 1984) ■ Norbeck Social Support Questionnaire (Norbeck, Lindsey, & Carrieri, 1981) ■ Baltimore Therapeutic Equipment (Kennedy & Bhambhani, 1991) ■ Nottingham Extended Activities of Daily Living Skills (Gladman, Lincoln, & Adams, 1993) ■ Driver performance testing ■ Structured observation of activity performance
Performance Skills	■ Motor and praxis skills	■ AMPS (Fischer, 1995)
	Praxis	■ Goodglass Test of Apraxia (Goodglass & Kaplan, 1972)
	Postural control/balance	■ Functional Reach Test (Duncan, Weiner, Chandler, & Studenski, 1990) ■ Tinetti Test (Tinetti, 1986) ■ Berg Balance Scale (Berg, Wood-Dauphinee, Williams, & Gayton, 1989) ■ Abreu's Quadraphonic Approach Postural Test (Abreu, 1994) ■ Motor Assessment Scale (MAS): Balance Items (Carr, Shepherd, Nordholm, & Lynne, 1985)

	Functional gross mobility
	  In bed
	  During seated task performance
	  Sit to stand
	  Functional ambulation
		■ MAS: Relevant items (Carr, Shepherd, Nordholm, & Lynne, 1985)
		■ Timed Get Up and Go Test (Mathias, Nayak, & Isscas, 1986)

(continued)

Table 1. Selected Assessments Used by Occupational Therapists With Stroke Survivors *(continued)*

Aspects of the Domain of Occupational Therapy	Specific Functions Within Each Aspect	Examples of Specific Assessments Used in Occupational Therapy Practice
	Skilled arm and hand function	■ Fugl-Meyer Assessment (Fugl-Meyer, Jaasko, Leyman, Olsson, & Steglind, 1975) ■ Wolf Motor Function Test (Morris, Uswatte, Crago, Cook, & Taub, 2001; Wolf et al., 2001) ■ MAS: Upper-limb items (Carr, Shepherd, Nordholm, & Lynne, 1985) ■ Arm Motor Assessment Test (Kopp et al., 1997) ■ Functional Test of Hemiplegic/Hemiparetic Upper Extremity (Wilson, Baker, & Craddock, 1984) ■ Chedoke Arm & Hand Activity Inventory (Barreca et al., 2004) ■ Motor Activity Log (Taub et al., 1993)
	■ Cognitive–perceptual Skills *Judgment* *Insight* *Memory* *Executive functions*	■ Loewenstein Occupational Therapy Cognitive Assessment (LOTCA; Katz, Itzkovich, Averbuch, & Elazar, 1989) ■ A-One (Arnadottir, 1990) ■ Contextual Memory Test (Toglia, 1993) ■ Rivermead Behavioral Memory Test (Malec, Zweber, & DePompolo, 1990)
	■ Communication/Social Skills	■ Functional assessment
Performance Patterns	■ Habits, routines, and rituals before onset of stroke ■ New habits and routines necessary to maintain health following stroke	■ Activity Card Sort (Baum & Edwards, 2008) ■ Client and family interview ■ Time configuration assessment
Contexts and Environments	■ Personal, physical, social, cultural, temporal, and virtual contexts and environments in which client is expected to perform activities and roles	■ COPM (Law et al., 1998) ■ Norbeck Social Support Questionnaire (Norbeck, Lindsey, & Carrieri, 1981) ■ Accessibility Checklist
Activity Demands	■ Physical, spatial, social, and temporal requirements of activities client wishes to/is expected to perform	■ Observational assessment during task performance ■ Interview
	■ Sensory–perceptual skills Spatial relations Visual scanning Visual perception	■ Motor-Free Visual Perception Test (MVPT; Colarusso & Hammill, 2003) ■ LOTCA (Katz, Itzkovich, Averbuch, & Elazar, 1989) ■ A-One (Arnadottir, 1990) ■ Cancellation tests (Diller et al., 1974)

Table 1. Selected Assessments Used by Occupational Therapists With Stroke Survivors *(continued)*

Aspects of the Domain of Occupational Therapy	Specific Functions Within Each Aspect	Examples of Specific Assessments Used in Occupational Therapy Practice

Client Factors	■ Primary Impairments
	   Flaccid paralysis
	      Paresis/weakness
		■ Fugel-Meyer Assessment (Fugel-Mayer et al., 1975)

	Spasticity	■ Ashworth Scale (Ashworth, 1964)
	Dysphagia	■ Videofluoroscopy ■ Modified barium swallow ■ Functional feeding assessment
	Somatosensory deficits	■ Screen of tactile and proprioceptive recognition ■ Screen of tactile discrimination ■ Stereognosis screen
	Visual field deficit *Unilateral visual inattention/spatial neglect* *Topographic disorientation* *Attention deficit*	■ Confrontation test ■ Cancellation tests ■ Functional assessment ■ Functional assessment—navigation ■ Test of Everyday Attention (Robertson, Ward, Ridgeway, & Nimmo-Smith, 1996)
	Impulsivity *Lability* *Impaired judgment* *Impaired insight*	■ Functional assessment

	■ Secondary Impairments
	   Postural malalignment
	      Pelvis, trunk, scapula, glenohumeral joint, forearm, wrist, hand
		■ Visual and manual postural assessment

	Limited flexibility between body segments Trunk, pelvis, scapula	■ Visual and manual assessment
	Limited passive range of motion	■ Goniometry
	Shoulder subluxation	■ Visual and manual assessment
	Upper-limb distal edema	■ Volumeter ■ Circumferential measurements ■ Figure-of-eight measurement (Pellecchia, 2004)
	Complex regional pain syndrome (formerly reflex sympathetic dystrophy)	■ Visual and manual assessment of symptoms
	Learned nonuse	■ Motor Activity Log (Taub et al., 1993)

to a healthy lifestyle and influence which goals will be most important to each stroke survivor. This area of assessment is less important than others during the acute phase after stroke because people have little control over their performance pattern in the hospital environment. However, evaluation of performance patterns becomes a priority during the rehabilitation phase and the phase of continuing adjustment. During these phases, the occupational therapist interviews the client and family members to determine relevant performance patterns before the stroke. For example, it is important for the occupational therapist to know how the person typically divided his or her time among work, self-care, and leisure activities. In addition, during the phase of continuing adjustment, it is important for the occupational therapist to determine what habits, routines, roles, and rituals the person has adopted after the stroke. In many cases, occupational therapy intervention to promote healthier performance patterns will play a significant role in preventing secondary impairments such as depression, limited range of motion, and learned nonuse.

Context and Environment

A core principle in occupational therapy is that performance is significantly influenced by the contexts in which people participate (AOTA, 2008b). Occupational therapists assess physical factors in the environment through accessibility assessments of clients' home, workplace, and community settings. Steps, entrances, and physical layout determine need for home adaptations and specialized equipment. Through interviews and interpersonal contact, occupational therapists also assess individualized factors in a person's cultural, personal, and social contexts. Temporal context, which includes a client's age and phase of stroke recovery, influences decisions about choice of evaluation tools and treatment interventions.

Activity Demands

When a stroke survivor has difficulties performing valued activities, the occupational therapist analyzes the specific activity demands that present challenges. The integrated results of assessing internal factors and activity demands inform the occupational therapist in determining how activities can be modified to facilitate performance or to provide feasible practice opportunities that may foster recovery of emerging skills.

After completing the occupational profile and determining which activities constitute a client's typical life pattern, the occupational therapist assesses the performance demands associated with each activity. There are two distinct purposes to this evaluation of activity demands. The more obvious purpose is to determine possible ways an activity might be adapted so that the stroke survivor will immediately be able to perform the task safely and independently, in spite of current impairments. This leads to recommendations for compensatory devices and strategies for self-care, leisure, and work activities. The second purpose for assessing activity demands is to determine how tasks can be manipulated for the purpose of providing practice opportunities for restoration and improvement of motor, cognitive, or perceptual skills. The process of activity analysis and subsequent activity grading (Radomski & Trombly Latham, 2008), a hallmark of occupational therapy intervention, has recently been termed "task-related training" (Dean & Shepherd, 1997; Thielman, Dean, & Gentile, 2004) and "repetitive task training" (French et al., 2007) in the rehabilitation literature.

Considerations in Assessment

Bottom-Up and Top-Down Approaches to Assessment

Occupational therapists consider each individual when determining whether to pursue a *bottom-up* or a *top-down* approach to evaluation (Holm, Rogers, & Stone, 2003). A bottom-up approach focuses on the client's generic abilities, with the rationale that impairments and abilities in client factors and skills will affect performance in an infinite number of present and future occupations. A top-down approach begins with an occupational profile and continues with a focused evaluation of client factors, performance skills, and performance patterns in the context of their impact on the client's capacity to perform valued activities and roles.

During the acute stage, a bottom-up assessment approach is advised. Because stroke survivors in the acute stage are adapting to their loss, and because it is virtually impossible to predict recovery levels, assessments of client factors are most critical. The resulting information enables occupational therapists to target intervention toward preventing secondary impairments, maximizing recovery, and making decisions for immediate discharge placement from the hospital setting.

During the rehabilitation stage, assessment is holistic and comprehensive. Occupational therapists dynamically move between top-down and bottom-up approaches. Determining the personal interests of a stroke survivor enables the therapist to observe performance in valued activities. Such observation provides the opportunity to assess the integration of skills, activity demands, and environmental context. In addition, continuous, detailed monitoring of client factors such as range of motion and postural alignment promotes the use of targeted interventions to prevent development of secondary impairments. Ongoing assessment of motor return, as well as skills in balance, reach, manipulation, and perceptual processing, ensures that interventions will provide appropriate challenges that enable clients to reach their maximal potential for recovery. Current reimbursement mechanisms in the United States encourage rehabilitation professionals to focus their assessment on immediate capacity to perform daily self-care activities, regardless of the recovery of motor or process skills. Although safety and independence are critical goals during the rehabilitation stage, therapists must not overlook the role of rehabilitation in maximizing the recovery of physical, cognitive, and perceptual function in each stroke survivor. Similarly, leisure and work activities may be more important to some stroke survivors than performance of self-care tasks. A person who continues to require assistance in putting on a shirt may well be an appropriate candidate for independent automobile driving or management of the family business.

Bottom-up assessments lose their significance during the stage of continuing adjustment when the emphasis is on improving quality of life and participation in a wide repertoire of meaningful roles. Even though stroke survivors maintain hope for continued recovery, a significant percentage must come to terms with creating a satisfying pattern of life activities in spite of residual losses in motor, cognitive, sensory, or perceptual function. Accordingly, assessments at this stage will focus on activities, contexts, and patterns of performance. Most important, assessments will determine how these factors can be integrated with the client's available skills to promote activity engagement and participation in valued occupations. Occupational therapy interventions after the acute and rehabilitation stages are targeted at the specific, immediate performance goals of a stroke survivor with the purpose of improving the person's overall quality of life. Pre- and post-intervention assessments of health quality of life can be useful in determining the impact of occupational therapy intervention during the stage of continuing adjustment.

Standardized and Observationally Based Assessments

Depending on the treatment setting and the purposes of assessment, occupational therapists determine whether to use standardized evaluations or non-standardized clinical observations of client performance in naturalistic contexts. Each type of assessment has its advantages and disadvantages, and occupational therapists are skilled in administering either category of client evaluation.

Standardized evaluations, when administered and scored according to published protocols, provide reliable and valid data for quantitative documentation of clients' progress. In addition, standardized evaluation scores can be used as outcome data for assessing the effectiveness of specific interventions. These assessments, however, may require significant time to administer. In addition, because consistent procedures must be followed on each administration, the evaluation context may fail to capture the environmental conditions under which the client will typically perform the skills or tasks being tested. Observationally based standardized assessments, such as the Assessment of Motor and Process Skills (AMPS) and Arnadottir Occupational Therapy Activities of Daily Living Neurobehavioral Evaluation (A-ONE), provide the benefits of standardized assessment while allowing for observation of behavior in naturalistic contexts.

During the acute stage after stroke, when the person's status may fluctuate from day to day and the priority is on implementing preventive interventions, occupational therapists rarely use standardized evaluations. During rehabilitation, however, occupational therapists routinely administer standardized evaluations to establish baseline data on admission to the facility. Periodic reevaluations determine an individual client's progress, influence continued treatment and discharge decisions, and provide data for program evaluation. Occupational therapy during the stage of continuing adjustment relies on standardized evaluations to determine clients' eligibility for demanding occupations such as driving or return to work. In addition, periodic standardized assessments during this time, when the natural course of recovery has typically subsided, are critical for determining intervention efficacy.

Boxes 2, 3, and 4 present case studies illustrating the occupational therapy evaluation and intervention process.

Box 2. Case Study: Acute Phase of Stroke

Paula Swift, an 81-year-old woman with a history of hypertension and diabetes mellitus, arrived at her local emergency room 5 hours after an acute onset of weakness in her left arm and leg. She had fallen at home while trying to get out of bed. When she did not answer the telephone for her daughter's routine morning call, her daughter asked the next-door neighbor to check on Ms. Swift. After finding her, the neighbor called 911 and paramedics took her to the hospital.

The stroke unit admitted Ms. Swift that afternoon, and doctors implemented conservative treatment and symptom management for an infarct in the right middle cerebral artery. The neurologist referred Ms. Swift for occupational therapy and physical therapy.

Ron Mills, the occupational therapist, first visited Ms. Swift the following afternoon. Her daughter and son-in-law were in the room with her. During the first occupational therapy visit, Ms. Swift was able to move her fingers and bend her elbow, but she felt unsure about her ability to sit up in bed. Ron instructed Ms. Swift's daughter in basic principles of bed positioning to prevent edema, to protect her left shoulder, and to maintain postural alignment. In particular, Ron demonstrated how to place pillows to keep Ms. Swift's left scapula protracted, her glenohumeral joint biased toward lateral rotation, her left hip from falling into either lateral or medial rotation, her knee slightly flexed, and her ankle in 90° dorsiflexion. After establishing baseline vital signs, Ron helped Ms. Swift sit on the side of her hospital bed. A quick check for signs of orthostatic hypotension was negative.

While Ms. Swift sat up with moderate physical support from Ron, the two of them chatted about Ms. Swift's family, neighborhood, and previous career as a bookkeeper. Ron casually asked about objects around the hospital room and hypothesized that Ms. Swift was demonstrating signs of left visual neglect. After describing visual neglect to Ms. Swift and her daughter, Ron advised the daughter to encourage family members to approach Ms. Swift from the left side in an effort to stimulate her attention to the left visual field.

The next day, when Ron returned for another session, Ms. Swift could no longer move her fingers. A quick motor screen revealed flaccid paralysis throughout her left arm and leg, but with sparing of trapezius, pectoralis major, and biceps brachii muscles.

Box 2. Case Study: Acute Phase of Stroke *(continued)*

Ron taught Ms. Swift to sit up on the side of the bed using her left arm for some support. Ms. Swift achieved this with minimal assistance from the therapist. Using a stool for foot support, Ms. Swift could sit independently. Ron challenged Ms. Swift's sitting balance by asking her to retrieve selected items from the top drawer of her bedside table. Ms. Swift used her outstretched left arm to provide some support to her sitting. Monitoring of vital signs revealed that Ms. Swift was stable throughout the activity. While Ms. Swift was engaged in this seated activity, Ron chatted with her about her hopes for returning home and asked questions about the layout and accessibility of her house.

Ron returned to Ms. Swift's room that afternoon, and provided instructions and assisted Ms. Swift in standing and transferring to a bedside chair. While Ms. Swift sat in the bedside chair, Ron taught her an exercise to maintain scapular mobility.

Next, Ron administered a feeding evaluation to Ms. Swift. Assessment of facial and oral tactile sensation and motor function revealed moderate tactile loss and mild weakness on the left side of the jaw, tongue, cheek, and lip muscles. Ron asked Ms. Swift to feed herself a bolus of applesauce while he auscultated her neck with a stethoscope. On hearing strong esophageal closure during the swallow and no subsequent abnormal sounds, Ron asked Ms. Swift to count to 10 out loud. Satisfied with Ms. Swift's ability to swallow a bolus of pureed consistency, Ron proceeded with a bolus of banana and then a small piece of soft bread. He continued the dysphagia evaluation for liquids and concluded that Ms. Swift now was a candidate for thickened liquids and a pureed diet.

On Ms. Swift's third morning on the stroke unit, Ron assisted her in transferring to a wheelchair and then in transferring from the wheelchair to the toilet. After Ms. Swift moved her bowels and cleaned herself, Ron helped her stand in front of the bathroom sink. He had arranged a comb, a soap dispenser, a washcloth, Ms. Swift's dentures, and Ms. Swift's lipstick along the sink's ledge. Ron instructed Ms. Swift to wash her face and comb her hair. As she did, he noticed that she was not attending to items on the left. She also was partially supporting herself by placing her right forearm on the sink's ledge. After the session, Ron documented that Ms. Swift would be an appropriate candidate for inpatient rehabilitation following her hospital disharge.

Ron visited Ms. Swift that afternoon for 15 minutes. During this session, Ms. Swift transferred to the bedside chair and demonstrated how she performed the scapular mobility exercise. With a rolling table positioned in front of her, Ron taught Ms. Swift to place her left arm on the table and to check systematically whether she could perform any specific shoulder, elbow, or hand movements. Ron instructed her in practicing flexion and extension of her elbow by using her left hand to apply skin lotion to her right forearm and hand.

Ms. Swift remained on the stroke unit for 5 days, after which she was discharged to a subacute inpatient rehabilitation facility located near her daughter's home. On Ms. Swift's fourth and fifth days on the stroke unit, therapy visits consisted of graded challenges to her sitting balance, standing balance, and visual scanning. These activities were complemented by exercises designed to maintain muscle length and joint alignment.

Daily feeding sessions consisted of instruction and practice in maintaining an optimal feeding posture; doing lip, jaw, and tongue exercises; and using compensatory strategies to minimize Ms. Swift's tendencies toward pocketing food in her cheek and drooling on the left side. With dysphagia intervention, Ms. Swift progressed to a mechanical soft diet and liquids of nectar consistency.

During each session, Ron answered Ms. Swift's questions about her prognosis with honest yet hopeful responses. Ms. Swift and her family left the hospital feeling optimistic about Ms. Swift's ability to regain function and skill performing daily-living tasks during her next phase of rehabilitation. Ms. Swift took a written copy of Ron's name and telephone number to share with her occupational therapist at the rehabilitation facility.

Box 3. Case Study: Rehabilitation Phase of Stroke

Jong-Su Kim had always been proud of his perseverance and discipline. After immigrating to the United States from Korea as a teenager, he quickly adapted to his new culture, excelled in school, and enjoyed a successful career as an elementary school principal. He retired only 3 years ago, and already he was developing an admirable golf game.

Mr. Kim also was proud of his attention to good health. Except for a history of hypertension, he was fit and active. When he experienced transient numbness in his left hand, he ignored it. Several days later, when he felt intermittent stiffness in his left arm and hand, he dismissed it as muscle soreness from playing with his grandchildren the previous weekend. The next day, though, after Mr. Kim lost his balance and fell, his wife took him to the emergency room at the local hospital. A computerized tomography (CT) scan revealed a right basal ganglia infarct, and the emergency room doctors began conservative treatment with anticoagulation medication.

After 5 days of hospitalization for acute stroke, Mr. Kim was admitted to a rehabilitation center. The initial occupational therapy evaluation, administered in two sessions on the first and second days of Mr. Kim's rehabilitation stay, included the Functional Independence Measure™ (FIM™); sensory testing of his left arm; a vision questionnaire and a vision screen; cognitive assessments, including the Contextual Memory Test and the Toglia Category Assessment; and motor assessments, including evaluation of sitting balance, standing balance, bed mobility, postural alignment during sitting and standing, and left-arm movement. During his first week at the rehabilitation facility, Mr. Kim's wife completed a home accessibility questionnaire, which gathered information about exterior and interior entrances, layout (with particular emphasis on the bathroom and the kitchen), and critical measurements.

The initial occupational therapy evaluation revealed that postural alignment in sitting was marked by excessive posterior pelvic tilt, which Mr. Kim could easily correct with cuing. Function in his right arm (the dominant one) was within normal limits, with normal strength and range of motion. He could maintain sitting balance with minimal challenges and moderate excursions. He could maintain standing only with contact guard and was unable to remain standing during attempts to shift his body weight in any direction. Although he did not report any problems on the vision questionnaire, functional testing revealed a mild impairment in ocular scanning. Cognitive assessments revealed that his orientation and memory were intact but that he had mild impairments in mental flexibility, concrete thinking, and impulsivity. Sensory testing revealed intact thermal, tactile, and proprioceptive sensation throughout his left arm, but mild distal impairments in his left leg. FIM testing of activities of daily living (ADLs) abilities revealed that he needed assistance for all self-care tasks, with greatest difficulty in bathing, dressing, toileting, and toilet transfer (see Table 2). Mr. Kim required minimal assistance for all bed mobility tasks and moderate assistance for stand–pivot transfers between his wheelchair and hospital bed.

In his left arm, Mr. Kim demonstrated full passive range of motion and preliminary movements as follows: He could elevate and retract his scapula through partial range and flex his shoulder at the glenohumeral joint through half-range against gravity, but with associated compensations of glenohumeral external rotation, scapular elevation, elbow flexion, and trunk lateral flexion to the right side. Mr. Kim was able to flex the fingers of his left hand as a single unit through the full range and extend the fingers as a single unit through three-fourths range. However, when he tried to hold a large cup, he could not modulate the pressure of his grasp. Mr. Kim was not able to use any of the available movements in his left arm during functional performance, and he relied exclusively on his intact right arm and hand during all ADLs. He was extremely motivated to improve his physical function so that he could return to his home to independently care for himself and participate in an active social life with his wife, friends, children, and grandchildren.

The primary treatment goals of occupational therapy were to improve Mr. Kim's sitting and standing balance, improve his motor control of his left arm, incorporate his left arm into functional activities, and regain his independ-

Box 3. Case Study: Rehabilitation Phase of Stroke *(continued)*

Table 2. Case Study: FIM Scores

	Initial Evaluation	Midterm Evaluation	Discharge Evaluation
Feeding	5	5	6
Personal hygiene	4	5	6
Bathing	3	4	5
Dressing: upper body	3	5	6
Dressing: lower body	2	5	6
Toileting	3	4	5
Toilet transfer	3	4	5
Social interaction	6	7	7
Problem solving	5	6	6

Scores range from 1 to 7.
1: Total assistance
2: Maximal assistance
3: Moderate assistance
4: Minimal contact assistance
5: Supervision or setup
6: Modified independence (no helper is needed; person uses an assistive device)
7: Total independence

ence in self-care tasks. Additional goals were to improve his oculomotor scanning and executive cognitive functions to levels before the stroke.

Mr. Kim participated in daily occupational therapy sessions 5 days per week, often accompanied by his wife. He also participated in a full physical therapy program that focused on regaining motor control in his leg and achieving independent gait. In addition, he attended biweekly sessions with a psychologist, with whom he discussed his anxieties related to the stroke and developed relaxation strategies for coping with this major life challenge.

Mr. Kim regularly attended recreation programs in the evenings and on the weekends. He particularly enjoyed participating in discussions about current events.

During his third week at the rehabilitation facility, Mr. Kim attended a five-session stroke education and wellness group. This multidisciplinary program was coordinated by occupational therapists at the rehabilitation center.

Occupational therapy intervention began with instruction to Mr. Kim and his wife in the key components of postural alignment while lying in bed and when sitting. Tina Clement, his occupational therapist, taught them a daily routine of stretching exercises with emphasis on promoting scapular and pelvic mobility. Mr. Kim became an active participant in preventing secondary impairments associated with immobility and in monitoring himself for any changes in his ability to move his left arm or hand. During daily sessions, Mr. Kim learned to shift weight in all planes while sitting and standing, and to use his left arm to support his body weight. At each session, Tina structured activities that would challenge Mr. Kim's current levels of balance, alignment, and left-arm movement. Mr. Kim left each session with a specific homework assignment to use a newly emerging motor skill in a functional context.

During the first week, Tina began every session with a quick check of how Mr. Kim was performing scapula-mobility and weight-bearing exercises, providing manual and verbal feedback when corrections were needed. During biweekly bedside sessions, Tina challenged Mr. Kim to apply newly emerging skills to his performance of self-care tasks and taught him compensatory strategies when appropriate.

(continued)

Box 3. Case Study: Rehabilitation Phase of Stroke *(continued)*

Tina conducted formal reevaluations on two occasions during Mr. Kim's 3-week hospitalization: at midterm and at discharge. At the midterm evaluation, Mr. Kim had made significant gains toward all occupational therapy goals. He had improved in virtually every self-care area on the FIM (see Table 2). He was now beginning to stand while performing activities at the sink, but he still lacked confidence in standing during toileting. His oculomotor scanning had improved, as evidenced by enhanced performance on a paper-and-pencil cancellation task included on the initial evaluation's visuomotor screening.

Further, his left-arm function had improved as an assist, with some use during bilateral activities and with increased active range of motion throughout the shoulder, elbow, wrist, and hand. He could now flex his shoulder 150° and abduct 120° against gravity with no evidence of the compensatory movements displayed at the initial evaluation. He could perform isolated internal and external glenohumeral rotation through three-fourths range in a gravity-eliminated plane. At the elbow, he now could flex against gravity (with no associated movements at other joints) through three-fourths range and could extend through the full range against gravity. Mild, fluctuating hypertonicity in his elbow flexors was modulated through routine self-stretching and nighttime wearing of a neuro hand splint, which maintained his finger joints in relaxed extension, kept his thumb extended, and kept his wrist extended to 15°. Mr. Kim now could supinate and pronate his forearm through three-fourths range.

Gains in hand function were also significant. Mr. Kim could flex and partially extend his wrist in a gravity-eliminated plane. He had regained full active range of motion for finger flexion in digits 1, 3, and 4, but still lacked complete flexion motion in digits 2 and 5. He adducted and abducted his thumb at the carpometacarpal joint through partial range. He exhibited early signs of individual finger movements and could slowly perform serial thumb opposition to each finger.

Functionally, Mr. Kim could use gross grasp to pick up and hold objects during grooming, feeding, and dressing tasks and to hold and squeeze toothpaste onto a toothbrush without assistance. He had learned to harness his emerging hand movements to achieve a weak pincer grasp, which he consistently used to take a shirt sleeve off his right arm when undressing. With training from Tina, he achieved the capacity to grasp a cup of water and slide it off the table with his left hand, then add his right hand to bring the cup bilaterally to his mouth to drink. Mr. Kim had made remarkable progress in awareness and incorporation of his left upper limb during task performance, but at the midpoint of his inpatient rehabilitation, he required verbal supervision to achieve maximal use of that arm and hand during ADLs.

At the midterm evaluation conference, Tina reported that Mr. Kim was now independent in bed mobility and could perform stand transfers with minimal assistance. The physical therapist reported that he was able to walk 20 feet on a level indoor surface with contact guard assistance and an ACE® wrap on his left ankle. He had progressed from using a quad cane to using no ambulation device. However, to compensate for persisting weakness in his left tibialis anterior, the physical therapist had ordered a customized ankle–foot orthosis.

At discharge, Mr. Kim had made further gains in all areas of occupational therapy intervention. He had achieved independence in self-care activities with either an assistive device (FIM score of 6) or supervision or setup (FIM score of 5). His standing balance and tolerance now were sufficient for independent toileting and sink activities. Mr. Kim continued to practice oculomotor scanning exercises and, wearing his prestroke reading glasses, he could read newspapers, magazines, and books. Through problem-solving practice with role-playing scenarios involving paying bills and planning a home renovation, he developed strategies for approaching complex situations with logic, flexibility, and a step-by-step approach.

Box 3. Case Study: Rehabilitation Phase of Stroke *(continued)*

Function in his left upper limb continued to improve with increases in active range of motion for glenohumeral flexion (now 170°), abduction (now 150°), and internal and external rotation (now full in a gravity-eliminated plane). He maintained his ability to extend his elbow fully and to pronate his forearm while increasing active range of motion in elbow flexion and forearm supination to three-fourths range against gravity. He had progressed to actively extending his wrist through three-fourths range in a gravity-eliminated plane, and he could flex and extend all his fingers through full range of motion.

Further, Mr. Kim showed beginning ability to abduct and adduct his fingers, had increased his capacity to perform thumb movements, and had increased the speed and accuracy of serial thumb opposition to each finger. Most important, he had improved his functional repertoire of using his left upper limb during task performance. For example, he now used his left hand for all dressing activities, including shoelace tying, and could stabilize food with a fork held in his left hand while cutting. He continued to wear a hand splint at night.

Mr. Kim returned home with his wife, with orders in place for home care occupational therapy and physical therapy. His wife was ready to arrange for installation of grab bars in the bathroom after a home care occupational therapist assessed Mr. Kim's needs. A tub seat and handheld shower spray, which Mr. Kim had practiced using during inpatient rehabilitation, were ordered before discharge. He was confident about navigating the four steps at the entrance to his ranch-style house, as he had practiced step-climbing in physical therapy sessions. He had received his customized ankle–foot orthosis but continued to require contact guard assistance during ambulation. He could easily enter and exit his family car, and he hoped to resume driving in time .

Mr. Kim was proud of the progress he had made during his 3-week inpatient rehabilitation program. Since he now met criteria for outpatient participation in a constraint-induced movement therapy program, he was considering this as a future option. With the goals of continuing to improve his motor skills and gradually resuming his family, social, and leisure roles, he looked forward to participating in home-based therapy and subsequent outpatient rehabilitation.

Box 4. Case Study: Continuing Adjustment Phase of Stroke

"I think I have a referral for you."

This was not the first time that Jan Lawson, an occupational therapist and certified hand therapist, had called Sandra Macey, an occupational therapist specializing in the area of neurorehabilitation, with information about a client who might benefit from Sandra's expertise. Eleanor Bolton, Jim's wife, had called Jan's office to inquire about occupational therapy to "get back some use in Jim's right arm." She explained that 5 years earlier, at age 77, Jim Bolton had a stroke that left him with paralysis in his right arm and problems speaking. After 6 weeks of inpatient rehabilitation and 8 weeks of home-based therapy, Mr. Bolton and his wife were left on their own.

Mr. Bolton continued to see a neurologist who gave him Botox injections every 3 months and a cardiologist who monitored his risk factors for another stroke. According to Mrs. Bolton, her husband had "been in a funk" for quite a long time but was vigilant about taking medications and watching his diet. Lately he was feeling more hopeful, and he wanted to do something to get back to his "old self." In addition, Mrs. Bolton had read a magazine article about brain plasticity and was hoping that Mr. Bolton could benefit from therapy to "help him move better."

Jan explained that her practice specialized in helping people who were recovering from orthopedic hand injuries, but she asked Mrs. Bolton if she and her husband would be interested in private-pay home-based services from Sandra. Mrs. Bolton replied that she'd be interested in meeting Sandra at their home.

Arriving at the Bolton's apartment, Sandra was pleased that they had gathered the written discharge summaries from Mr. Bolton's stay in a subacute rehabilitation facility as she had requested. After introducing herself, she quickly reviewed the information, noting that Mr. Bolton was a retired salesman who had been active in his community church and Rotary Club. He had sustained an infarct to his right middle cerebral artery, with subsequent hemiparesis, spasticity, Broca's aphasia, and ideomotor apraxia. When he left the rehabilitation facility, he could ambulate on indoor surfaces with a quad cane and an ankle orthosis, but needed to use a wheelchair for outdoor mobility. The Boltons had two grown children and five grandchildren, all of whom lived more than 500 miles away.

Sandra asked whether the Boltons remembered Mr. Bolton's occupational therapy treatment from 5 years ago. They replied that the therapy had been quite helpful in teaching him techniques to use the toilet and feed, bathe, and dress himself, but they were disappointed that he did not regain any function in his right arm or hand. Sandra was careful to point out that there was no guarantee she could help Mr. Bolton regain movement and that it was unlikely he would ever move his right arm the way he had before his stroke. However, after evaluating his motor skills, she could determine what small goals would be attainable. Further, she could help Mr. Bolton find ways to be active again.

Sandra asked the Boltons to record information on a time-configuration assessment about how Mr. Bolton spent his time on a typical day. She helped them fill in a few lines of the grid to make sure they understood the instructions. Sandra then asked Mr. Bolton what he wanted to do that he was unable to at that time. Mr. Bolton responded as best he could verbally and demonstrated how his right arm tightened into a flexed position when he walked. Sandra followed with a question, based loosely on the COPM, to find out the things Mr. Bolton did prior to his stroke that he wished he could do now.

Between the Bolton's responses, Sandra ascertained that Mr. Bolton had stopped going to church on Sundays, rarely left their apartment without Mrs. Bolton, and felt guilty that Mrs. Bolton had had to take over most of the responsibilities related to managing their household and maintaining communication with their children. In response to specific questions about self-care performance and safety, Sandra learned that Mr. Bolton was independent in feeding, dressing (except for some fasteners), and toileting. His bathroom was equipped with safety bars at the toilet and in the tub, and he had a tub seat and a handheld shower spray. He was independent in bathing but, for safety reasons, bathed only when Mrs. Bolton was nearby. On further questioning, Mrs. Bolton confided that Mr.

Box 4. Case Study: Continuing-Adjustment Phase of Stroke *(continued)*

Bolton sat for all toileting and sink activities because he was unsure of his standing balance. Sandra also learned that Mr. Bolton was self-conscious about a 15-pound paunch he had developed over the past few years.

Sandra's postural assessment included evaluation of Mr. Bolton's standing balance, weight-bearing ability, and weight-shifting ability in all directions. Following her assessment of Mr. Bolton's strategy in standing up and sitting down, she asked him to walk into his bedroom and lie down on his bed. Sandra then assessed him rolling to his right and left sides and sitting from a supine position. She assessed the muscle tone in his arms and legs and his ability to move each arm and leg while supine. They then returned to the dining room table, where Sandra evaluated Mr. Bolton's ability to follow multistep commands, his praxis and dexterity (using his left arm), and the movement potential in his right forearm and hand. Unfortunately, Mr. Bolton did not meet the minimum criteria to consider intervention using constraint-induced movement therapy, a treatment protocol with considerable evidence for efficacy in improving arm function in patients with mild hemiparesis.

Sandra concluded the session by telling the Boltons that she thought she could teach Mr. Bolton techniques to control his spasticity, improve his balance, and use his limited available right-arm movement to assist grossly in bilateral tasks. She shared her opinion that with occupational therapy intervention, Mr. Bolton could play a more active role in helping Mrs. Bolton manage the household and that, if he were interested, he could begin to engage safely in activities outside his apartment. The Boltons agreed to eight additional private-pay, home-based sessions once a week, with the first to occur 3 days later. When Sandra left, she reminded the Boltons to complete the time-configuration assessment before the next visit.

Sandra returned 3 days later with a small notebook to record Mr. Bolton's progress and homework assignments. A quick review of his responses to the time-configuration assessment confirmed her suspicions that he spent most of his time in the house watching television and was rarely engaged in activity that was socially meaningful, intellectually stimulating, or physically challenging.

Sandra began by teaching Mr. Bolton scapula-mobility exercises, writing the directions in his notebook and advising him to perform them five times every day. She then had him practice shifting his weight while sitting and standing and taught him a new way to stand up from and sit down in a chair, with an emphasis on distributing his body weight evenly over both legs. She drew a picture and described the technique in Mr. Bolton's notebook, and instructed him to consider using this technique whenever he stood up and sat down.

Next, Sandra suggested that they get the mail from the building's lobby. Mr. Bolton replied to the best of his ability that he could not hold the mail, pointing to his right arm and gesturing to the quad cane in his left hand. Sandra asked whether Mr. Bolton had any tote or plastic grocery bags. Mr. Bolton gestured below the sink; Sandra took out a bag and then instructed Mr. Bolton to carry the bag on his right forearm. Sandra and Mr. Bolton left the apartment.

In the hallway, Sandra asked Mr. Bolton to press the button to call the elevator. Mr. Bolton looked at Sandra with annoyance, pointing to his right hand, then his left hand and the cane. Sandra told Mr. Bolton to try to let go of the cane for a moment to press the button, reassuring him that she was right next to him. Mr. Bolton was surprised that he could maintain his standing balance while letting go of his cane. He tried this again when they were in the elevator, pressing the lobby button.

Once they were in the mailroom, Sandra saw that the mailbox was slightly lower than arm level, requiring Mr. Bolton to bend slightly to reach it. Sandra made a mental note to incorporate this type of weight shift into his balance exercises, and helped him open the box. She also helped him retrieve the mail and put it into the bag on his right arm and informed him that she could help him become able to do this by himself. Back in the apartment, Mr. Bolton removed the mail from the bag and placed it on the counter for Mrs. Bolton, sharing with her his surprise and pride at having successfully completed this task.

(continued)

Box 4. Case Study: Continuing-Adjustment Phase of Stroke *(continued)*

In a safe place next to Mr. Bolton's bed, Sandra taught him a new exercise, requiring him to bend and straighten his knees while standing. She used her hands to cue him for optimal position of his pelvis. She showed Mrs. Bolton how to supervise him in this exercise and described the exercise in his homework notebook. As Sandra left, she asked Mr. Bolton to practice the homework exercises. She also asked him to think about activities he would like to be able to perform and to identify two specific tasks he would like to practice with Sandra's help.

Sandra continued her sessions with Mr. Bolton for 8 weeks. The occupational therapy intervention combined exercises and activities to enhance Mr. Bolton's safety in standing, his flexibility between body segments, and his use of minimal right-arm movements during bilateral activities. After a few sessions, Mr. Bolton mastered the ability to go to the building lobby, open his mailbox, retrieve the mail, and bring it up to the apartment alone. He found that he enjoyed seeing his neighbors during this daily routine.

Following discussion, Mr. Bolton and Sandra identified two activity goals: to be able to water the plants in the apartment and to be able to write his name legibly with his left hand. To meet Mr. Bolton's goal of watering plants, Sandra helped him rearrange the locations of his plants so that he could safely reach them, and she arranged with Mrs. Bolton to leave a half-filled watering can on the window sill once a week. Next, Mr. Bolton practiced the necessary shifts in body weight to perform the task of watering each plant. At first, Sandra provided physical support, but she gradually decreased her assistance as Mr. Bolton gained confidence in maintaining his balance.

For the handwriting goal, Sandra brought a workbook of cursive-writing worksheets and instructed Mr. Bolton to sit in good alignment at the dining room table, with his right arm on the table holding down the paper. Sandra dated the sheets, assigning Mr. Bolton one sheet to complete every day. Over the weeks, Mr. Bolton was pleased to see that he was gaining better control of the pen and forming neater graphics. After 1 month, he was confident in signing his name and proudly signed greeting cards to family and friends.

At the fifth session, Sandra asked Mr. Bolton if he ever used the computer in the apartment's second bedroom. Although he had used a computer at his previous job, he never had time to use the family's computer, which was primarily used by Mrs. Bolton. After his stroke, he never considered the possibility of engaging in computer activities.

Sandra placed the mouse to the left side of the keyboard and instructed Mr. Bolton to use the same sitting posture he used during writing practice. Mr. Bolton attempted to use the mouse with his left hand. Sandra gave him the assignment of playing solitaire at least once every day to gain basic control of the mouse. Within 3 weeks, Mr. Bolton felt proficient at using the mouse. His reading comprehension was unimpaired, and he could follow directions to navigate Web sites and interactive games. Sandra introduced him to literature on options for one-handed typing, and Mr. Bolton selected a commercially available adapted keyboard.

At the end of the 8 weeks, Mr. Bolton had not regained any abilities to move his right arm or hand. However, he had improved his confidence and safety in standing and walking and was able to stand during toilet activities. He had established new daily routines of getting the mail, watering plants, using the computer, and performing stretching exercises to manage the spasticity in his right arm and leg. His children were delighted that he could send periodic e-mails to them, and he delighted in downloading photographs of his grandchildren.

In addition, Sandra had spent one session with Mr. Bolton and Mrs. Bolton practicing getting on and off a wheelchair-accessible bus that stopped one block from their home. Mr. Bolton was now considering going back to church, using his wheelchair and the bus to get there, leaving the wheelchair at the door, and walking inside the church.

Mr. Bolton thanked Sandra for her help. When he gave her a good-bye kiss on the last visit, he proudly indicated that he was back to doing some of the activities that were important to him and that he had never imagined would be possible after his stroke.

Intervention

Occupational therapy intervention with stroke survivors is a collaborative process between practitioner and client. The ultimate goals are engagement in a wide repertoire of personally meaningful occupations and a healthy lifestyle that supports independence, prevention of additional strokes, and prevention of secondary impairments. The intervention process consists of three components: (1) developing an intervention plan in which objective and measurable goals are established, with clear guidelines for treatment approaches, treatment personnel, and frequency and duration of service; (2) intervention implementation; and (3) intervention review.

Intervention Plan

As a part of the occupational therapy process, the occupational therapist develops an intervention plan that documents (1) the client's goals within an occupational framework, (2) the planned intervention approaches, and (3) recommendations or referrals to others. The intervention plan outlines and guides the therapist's actions and is based on the best available evidence to meet the identified outcomes (AOTA, 2008b).

Intervention Implementation

The broad goals of occupational therapy intervention with stroke survivors are to
- *Prevent* secondary impairments
- *Restore* performance skills
- *Modify* activity demands and the contexts in which activities are performed to support safe, independent performance of valued activities within the constraints of stroke-related fatigue and motor, cognitive, or perceptual limitations
- *Promote* a healthy and satisfying lifestyle that includes adherence to medication routine, appropriate diet, appropriate levels of physical activity, and satisfying levels of engagement in social relationships and activities

- *Maintain* performance and health that the stroke survivor has previously regained or the neuropathology has spared.

Tables 3–7 provide examples of occupational therapy intervention under the rubric of these five approaches.

Intervention to Prevent Secondary Impairments

Preventive occupational therapy intervention with stroke survivors seeks to minimize the risks of six kinds of secondary impairments:
- Abnormal changes in postural alignment (postural deformities)
- Pain associated with immobility or abnormal joint alignment
- Learned nonuse
- Injury due to falls
- Aspiration during feeding, eating, and swallowing
- Depression following stroke.

In each of these areas, occupational therapy intervention is part of a multidisciplinary effort with physicians, nurses, and other rehabilitation professionals.

Prevention of postural deformities. Intervention begins immediately following stroke with slow, gentle, passive stretch to all muscle groups. Mammalian muscles normally maintain their maximum length through passive stretch by antagonist muscles during the natural course of active daily movement. Immobility due to paralysis removes the natural course of repeated passive muscle stretch and leads to loss in muscle length (Buschbacher, 1996).

During the acute stage after stroke, occupational therapists instruct patients in using available motor control in the affected and nonaffected limbs to begin a self-exercise program designed to stretch muscles gently throughout the body (Langhorne & Pollock, 2002; Scottish Intercollegiate Guidelines Network, 2002). This regimen needs to be continued as a routine exercise program throughout the person's life. Since motor capabilities are likely to change with recovery and over time with aging, it is important that therapists review and modify the stretching program during subsequent stages of rehabilitation and continuing adjustment. For stroke survivors with more severe disabilities who never regain sufficient motor control to implement their own routine stretching programs, the occupational therapist teaches caregivers passive stretch regimens that are individually tailored to be both appropriate to the survivor's needs and feasible within the context of the caregiver's physical abilities and time demands. Feasibility and routine incorporation into daily patterns are key factors in adherence to any preventive health program. In addition, early adherence to bed and wheelchair positioning protocols (Gillen & Burkhardt, 2004) may prevent development of abnormal postural patterns, such as scapula retraction, thoracic kyphosis, or abnormalities in pelvic alignment.

Prevention of pain and other complications associated with immobility or abnormal joint alignment. All stroke survivors, at all stages of recovery, may experience pain. The causes of pain after stroke are associated with preventable, secondary impairments such as abnormal shoulder alignment, pressure ulcers, edema, and joint immobility.

Studies of stroke-associated shoulder pain consistently show that prevention is more effective than treatment (Snels et al., 2002; Vuagnat & Chantraine, 2003). If allowed to develop, adhesive capsulitis, rotator cuff tear, and chronic regional pain syndrome require extensive rehabilitation intervention and possible surgery, all with limited impact on patients' perceived pain.

Prevention of these secondary impairments requires continuous attention to maintain the appropriate kinesiological relationship between the scapula and the humerus of a paretic arm. In particular, the scapula must protract during shoulder flexion and must upwardly rotate during shoulder flexion or abduction beyond 90° (Bagg & Forrest, 1988; Bourne, Choo, Regan, MacIntyre, & Oxland, 2007; Freedman & Munro, 1966). Furthermore, external rotation of the humeral head must accompany end ranges of flexion and abduction (Stokdijk, Eilers, Nagels, & Rozing, 2003). This kinematic relationship, often referred to as *scapulohumeral rhythm* (Inman, Saunders, & Abbott,

1944), must be maintained at rest and during movement and handling by caregivers. The use of overhead pulley exercises by stroke survivors who do not exhibit scapulohumeral rhythm has been associated with higher risk of developing shoulder pain and should be avoided (Kumar, Metter, Mehta, & Chew, 1990).

Occupational therapy practitioners prevent secondary impairments associated with shoulder pain by teaching stroke survivors effective strategies for self-range of motion. Specifically, clients learn to achieve scapula mobility before attempting to perform active or passive motions at the glenohumeral joint (Gillen & Burkhardt, 2004). In addition, they learn to combine glenohumeral with scapular motions, especially when flexing the humerus beyond 90°. Occupational therapy practitioners also provide individualized training to caregivers on proper handling of the shoulder girdle.

Glenohumeral subluxation is commonly seen in hemiplegic clients. Although some studies conclude that subluxation is only one of several possible causes of shoulder pain following stroke (Bohannon & Andrews, 1990; Zorowitz, Hughes, Idank, Ikai, & Johnston, 1996), prevention of shoulder subluxation is an important focus of upper-limb rehabilitation after stroke (Ada, Foongchomcheay, & Canning, 2005) due to its association with poor upper-limb function (Hanger et al., 2000), pain (Paci, Nannetti, Taiti, Baccini, & Rinaldi, 2007), and reflex sympathetic dystrophy (Dursun, Dursun, Ural, & Cakci, 2000). Occupational therapists assess the specific type of glenohumeral subluxation and provide a variety of interventions, depending on the type and the severity of misalignment. Interventions include provision of external supports (Ada, Foongchomcheay, & Canning, 2005) and electrical stimulation to rotator cuff muscles (Vuagnat & Chantraine, 2003). At present, the evidence is insufficient to support the routine provision of either of these two interventions (Ada, Foongchomcheay, & Canning, 2005; New Zealand Guidelines Group, 2003; Price & Pandyan, 2000).

Hand edema, another secondary impairment, is associated with immobility, a dependent position of the hand, and limited natural pumping of extracellular fluid associated with active muscle contraction. First and foremost, occupational therapists prevent hand edema by encouraging active movement of the hand for those clients who have the motor capacity. For those clients who are unable to actively contract the muscles of the hand, positioning to elevate the hand, as well as compression and gentle massage techniques, are recommended interventions (Gillen & Burkhardt, 2004). Use of continuous passive motion technology (Dirette & Hinojosa, 1994) or neuromuscular stimulation (Faghri et al., 1994) in conjunction with elevation of the hand is more effective than elevation alone in reducing edema immediately following stroke (Geurts, Visschers, van Limbeek, & Ribbers, 2000).

Pressure ulcers are associated with prolonged immobility. Stroke survivors who fail to achieve the capacity to shift body weight when sitting, or to change their position in bed, are at risk of developing this painful and costly secondary impairment. Stroke survivors who establish daily routines involving movement and frequent adjustment of body weight off bony prominences have little risk of developing pressure ulcers. Therefore, prevention is achieved through the early introduction of activity-based interventions designed to enhance the abilities of stroke survivors to move about in bed and to maintain sitting balance when shifting their center of mass throughout all possible permutations of the three cardinal planes (Mudie, Winzeler-Mercay, Radwan, & Lee, 2002).

Prevention of learned nonuse. Beyond the constraints imposed by secondary mechanical impairments, many stroke survivors demonstrate "learned nonuse" (Kunkel et al., 1999; Mark & Taub, 2004). This phenomenon describes the common situation in which a person fails to use his or her paretic arm, even when muscle activity and sensory awareness are available. The phenomenon of learned nonuse was first observed in neuroscience research studies in which the motor recovery of laboratory animals was observed after experimentally induced lesions to one cerebral hemisphere (Taub, 1976). With available sensorimotor function in one remaining forelimb and hindlimb, the experimental animals quickly learned to compensate for their temporary loss of function in the paretic limbs. When researchers prevented this compensatory reliance on the spared limbs through external restraint in the form of plaster casts, the animals exhibited enhanced recovery of the paretic limbs.

Similar to the laboratory animals in research studies, a primary explanation for the phenomenon of learned nonuse is that early after brain injury, stroke survivors learn to rely exclusively on their unaffected limbs for activity performance. Even when motor abilities begin to reemerge with neural recovery, a person finds that it is more efficient to continue performing tasks with the unaffected arm and leg, and significant effort is required to incorporate the paretic limbs into task performance.

Learned nonuse begins a negative spiral of events. Without active use, the paretic limbs are more vulnerable to developing secondary impairments associated with immobility, such as limited range of motion and edema. Furthermore, practice opportunities with the affected limbs, which are essential to neural reorganization following brain injury, are lost if the person does not attempt to use the paretic arm or leg during functional activities. The theory of learned nonuse may explain why upper-limb recovery often lags behind recovery of function in the paretic lower limb. Whereas each attempt to stand or walk requires bilateral activity in the legs, many upper-limb activities may be accomplished by using the unaffected side exclusively.

During the acute and rehabilitation stages after stroke, prevention of learned nonuse is a primary goal in occupational therapy intervention. Therapists use every opportunity to teach the stroke survivor to be aware of and to use the paretic limbs to the limits of current available motor function. Using the paretic leg and arm to support body weight, called "weightbearing" in some literature (Howle, 2002), is usually the first tangible way a stroke survivor can learn to rely on his or her hemiparetic limbs and to reincorporate them into his or her overall body schema. Activities requiring the person to shift body weight in a variety of directions may also play a role in preventing learned nonuse by challenging the stroke survivor to be aware of and use muscles on the paretic side.

To prevent learned nonuse in the paretic arm, therapists continually assess motor potential in specific muscles, using external support or special positioning to detect emerging changes. In addition, occupational therapists teach patients to understand movement linkages and to check actively for changes in their ability to recruit specific muscles. Therapy sessions become opportunities for stroke survivors to share their discoveries with their therapists. In turn, occupational therapists structure activities that enable patients to practice emerging movement capacities. For a clinical example of this intervention, see Case Study: Rehabilitation Phase of Stroke (Box 3).

Prevention of injury due to falls. Occupational therapy practitioners provide interventions to reduce both intrinsic and extrinsic risk factors for falling. Intrinsic client factors in the stroke population include muscle weakness, balance impairments, and attention impairments. Occupational therapy practitioners work with clients in the acute and rehabilitation stages of stroke recovery to provide them with opportunities to practice unsupported sitting and functional standing. In the context of functional activity performance, stroke survivors develop strategies for adjusting to shifts in their body's center of mass to enhance their balance skill and efficacy. To reduce fear of falling and to ensure more favorable outcomes if falls do occur, it is critical that stroke survivors have opportunities for supervised practice performing bathroom and other household activities, as well as getting themselves back into an upright position from the floor.

Extrinsic risk factors for falls among stroke survivors can be significantly reduced through assessment of the home environment and introduction of structural adaptations designed to meet individual needs for external supports for stability in the bathroom, kitchen, bedroom, and other living spaces. Multifaceted interventions by occupational therapists with elderly people in the community have been shown to be effective in reducing the risk of falls and related injuries (Clemson et al., 2004).

Prevention of aspiration during feeding, eating, and swallowing. Dysphagia—difficulty eating and swallowing due to motor or cognitive impairments—is common immediately following stroke, but often subsides after the acute stage of recovery (Smithard et al., 1997). In acute stroke care settings, occupational therapists are members of the professional team that provides evaluation and intervention to prevent aspiration during feeding. Initially, the occupational therapist assesses oral motor skills and swallowing efficiency to help the physician determine when the client may proceed from alternative feeding to a specified sequence of solid and liquid food consistencies. Earliest solids are purees, followed by semi-solids, soft solids, chewable foods, and, finally, foods with multiple textures. Earliest liquids are spoon-thick, followed by honey-thick, nectar-thick, and, finally, thin liquids.

When a client is cleared for oral intake, occupational therapists provide positioning intervention to ensure that the client's seated posture contributes to safe and efficient swallowing. In addition, occupational therapists use techniques to improve sensation, strength, and muscle tone of oral structures to maximize the potential for safe, independent eating (AOTA, 2007d; Avery-Smith & Dellarosa, 1994).

Similar interventions may be indicated after the acute stage for clients who continue to demonstrate continued feeding impairments. These individuals are most typically seen in nursing facilities or are living at home with significant levels of caregiver assistance.

Prevention of depression following stroke. Close to half of all stroke survivors are diagnosed with depression within the first year following stroke (Anderson, Hackett, & House, 2004). Debate continues as to whether depression after a stroke is an organic result of a stroke's neuropathology or a secondary reaction to the catastrophic losses and life changes associated with stroke (Turner-Stokes, 2003). Occupational therapists play two important roles in preventing depression after a stroke: First, through their close contact with stroke survivors, occupational therapists can recognize signs and symptoms of depression and communicate with other health professionals to ensure that clients receive appropriate medical and psychological intervention. Second, by promoting independence, autonomy, participation, and hope for the future, occupational therapists can reduce the overwhelming emotional burdens of adjusting to life after a stroke. The need for participation in valued life roles continues through the entire life of a stroke survivor. For this reason, stroke survivors should have continued access to targeted occupational therapy interventions designed to promote task performance when there are changes in their interests, family supports, or living environment.

For examples of interventions to prevent secondary impairments, see Table 3.

Intervention to Restore Performance Skills

Neuroscience research is yielding increasing evidence that stroke survivors are capable of redeveloping lost skills through therapeutic practice (Butefisch, 2004; Johansen-Berg et al., 2002). Occupational therapy provides stroke survivors with structured practice opportunities to maximize emerging skills. Doing this is not nearly as simple as it sounds. When people practice maladaptive strategies, they learn patterns of behavior that may be counterproductive to future improvements in functional performance. To provide appropriate practice opportunities, therapists must clearly envision the intended practice outcomes and skillfully manipulate a variety of factors during each practice session. These factors include instructions, feedback, activity parameters, salient conditions in the practice environment, and practice schedules. The ultimate goal is for clients to generalize their new skills to enhanced performance of activities in their daily lives.

Motor skills include the abilities to maintain balance and postural alignment during activity performance in sitting and standing postures and to use the paretic arm and leg for functional tasks. A person's level of functional motor skills is influenced by the interaction among several factors:

- The degree of physiological damage to neural structures
- The person's inherent capacity for neural reorganization

- The extent to which secondary impairments impose mechanical or other constraints on the person's ability to move
- The person's ability to recognize newly emerging capacities for movement and to apply emerging motor potential to practical use in functional task performance.

The degree of physiological damage to neural structures is determined at the time of the stroke by the infarct or hemorrhage itself and the medical management of its acute sequelae. The mechanism for neural reorganization is only partially understood. Current research indicates that with sufficient and appropriate environmental challenges, brain regions previously unassociated with particular functions can assume new roles (Johansen-Berg et al., 2002). This mechanism may be similar to the development of new skills in healthy people (Asanuma & Pavlides, 1997). Environmental challenges, however, require the expertise of an occupational therapist who can assess each person's ongoing changes in motor potential and understand the kinesiological foundations of efficient movement strategies. The occupational therapist designs tasks that challenge emerging movement capacities without promoting the development of secondary impairments that may constrain a person's potential to develop functional motor skills.

The most common secondary impairments limiting stroke survivors from using their full emerging motor potential are the loss in muscle length due to spasticity or immobility in selected muscles; changes in postural alignment; difficulties in linking or unlinking motions of adjacent body segments, such as the scapula and humerus, scapula and thorax, or pelvis and lumbar spine; and learned nonuse.

Cognitive skills include the abilities to attend to environmental stimuli; remember relevant information; plan, organize, and sequence activity performance; and assess actions. *Perceptual skills* include the abilities to interpret sensory information and navigate the spatial environment. Cognitive and perceptual deficits are often viewed collectively as neurobehavioral impairments. Both are neural sequelae to brain injury that affect a person's functional behaviors.

Table 3. Examples of Interventions to Prevent Secondary Impairments

Focus of Intervention	Desired Result	Sample Strategy
Client factors	Prevent loss of flexibility in paralyzed muscles	Teach client daily routine of individualized stretching (by client or caregiver) Establish optimal postural alignment while in bed, while sitting, and while standing
	Prevent injury due to falls	Provide interventions to improve balance strategies Provide interventions to enhance safety and efficiency in sit-to-stand wheelchair transfers and functional ambulation
	Prevent aspiration during self-feeding	Provide individualized positioning to ensure optimal posture during feeding Provide interventions to develop oral–motor skills
Motor skill	Prevent learned nonuse	Encourage early use of the paretic arm during functional activities to each patient's current potential Adapt activities to provide opportunities to use newly emerging movement recovery
Context	Prevent injury due to falls	Assess living environment for environmental hazards and recommend home modifications (e.g., tub seat and handheld shower spray, safe use of floor coverings, safety bars in bathroom)
Performance patterns	Prevent depression	Provide interventions that enable client to develop activity patterns providing sense of self-efficacy and meaningful engagement

Specific cognitive and perceptual impairments after stroke are determined by the extent and the location of brain pathology. For example, right parietal lesions are typically associated with visuospatial deficits, such as unilateral neglect and disturbed topographical orientation; left frontal lobe pathology is associated with dysfunction in producing language or sequencing activities (e.g,, not following the order of steps in preparing a meal or getting dressed). The severity of neurobehavioral deficits ranges from mild sequelae, in which a person experiences difficulty only with complex, instrumental activities in the work environment, to severe impairments that affect a person's capacity to perform basic self-care tasks.

Occupational therapy intervention for stroke survivors with cognitive and perceptual impairments begins with structured assessment (see Table 1) to determine the following:

- Their level of self-awareness of the neurobehavioral deficit that they exhibit during task performance, which will critically affect the person's capacity to improve skills or apply compensatory strategies
- Their potential to improve impaired skills through structured, graded practice
- Their potential to apply new strategies that might facilitate compensation for cognitive or perceptual deficits.

On the basis of their findings from these assessments, occupational therapists develop individualized treatments designed to accomplish the following goals:

- Enhance clients' awareness of their neurobehavioral impairments
- Provide clients with graded practice opportunities to improve specific skills that are amenable to change
- Enable clients to assess their own activity performance to make decisions that will enhance their success in performing specific tasks
- Teach clients alternative strategies to maximize their performance in task situations that present cognitive or perceptual challenges.

Unlike motor paralysis, disorders of cognition or perception are "invisible disabilities" associated with stroke. Both physiological and psychological factors may contribute to the common problem in stroke survivors of denying difficulties in processing information or organizing behaviors. However, survivors' awareness of deficits and effective appraisal of their own performance are key foundations for improving neurobehavioral skills and applying compensatory strategies to task performance. Through carefully selected activity challenges and guided questions before, during, and after task performance, occupational therapists help stroke survivors develop insight into their cognitive–perceptual assets and limitations (Katz, 2005).

Many stroke survivors exhibit significant potential to redevelop lost neurobehavioral skills through rigorous practice. The ultimate goal in this type of remedial intervention is for the client to generalize enhanced skill levels to performance of life activities. Using the well-supported educational principle that generalization of learning is best achieved through random practice of core, underlying, foundational skills (Giuffrida, Shea, & Fairbrother, 2002; Hall & Magill, 1995), patients practice targeted strategies in a variety of different tasks and environmental contexts. For example, if the goal is to improve skill in visual scanning, the client applies a core strategy of systematically moving his or her eyes horizontally from left to right in a series

of seemingly unrelated tasks. One task might require the person to find all the letter "M's" in several lines of printed text. Another task might require the person to select a designated command on the horizontal toolbar of repeated Web pages. In yet another task, the person might have to select a particular brand of breakfast cereal from a collection of cereal boxes arranged horizontally on several pantry shelves. Task difficulty is gradually increased by increasing the complexity in ways that are pertinent to the targeted skill. Since the amount of practice is a key factor in learning success (Schmidt & Lee, 2005), occupational therapy practitioners teach patients and their families ways to structure additional practice challenges outside therapy sessions.

Emotional coping skills include a core of effective strategies that stroke survivors must develop to negotiate their interactions with others and return to full participation in their communities. The emotional challenges of living with the sequelae of stroke are enormous. The physical difficulties of paralysis, impaired balance, and fatigue, often combined with difficulties processing information or communicating, significantly affect a person's core identity. Some stroke survivors may mourn lost roles, feel incompetent in performing routine activities, and feel embarrassed by their dependence on others. It may be difficult to return to social activities and to ask for help with tasks that were previously easy and automatic. In addition, it takes effort to plan one's day so that time will be used meaningfully, energy conserved, and environmental obstacles avoided.

Stroke survivors need opportunities to practice the skills that they will need to cope with the emotional challenges they face every day. Through role-playing and practice in real environments, such as at the bank, on the bus, and in the workplace, occupational therapists help stroke survivors begin to problem-solve. The goal is to develop day-to-day strategies that they can use in emotionally challenging situations. Occupational therapists design "homework" in which stroke survivors perform specific self-selected tasks and report the outcome in the next therapy session. Homework assignments and practice opportunities are geared toward each person's present and anticipated environmental contexts. Examples include calling an old friend for the first time, making a purchase at the nursing home's gift shop, paying a bill, and planning and taking a trip to the local mall. Research indicates that health-related quality of life after stroke relates more significantly to a person's social network and general emotional orientation than to the degree of physical recovery (Jonsson, Lindgren, Hallstrom, Norrving, & Lindgren, 2005).

The Evidence-Based Practice section of this Guideline provides support for the effectiveness of occupational therapy interventions to enhance skills in stroke survivors.

For examples of interventions to restore performance skills, see Table 4.

Table 4. Examples of Interventions to Restore Performance Skills

Focus of Intervention	Desired Result	Sample Strategy
Performance skills	Restore functional use of hemiparetic arm to maximum potential	Provide passive movement and exercise to improve scapulohumeral rhythm, followed by functional reaching tasks in all possible planes of motion Provide structured opportunities for client to practice performing functional tasks requiring highest level of available grasp patterns from variety of trunk and arm positions
	Restore functional sitting balance skills to maximum potential	Engage client in functional tasks requiring graded challenges to shifting weight in all planes of motion while sitting
	Restore functional standing balance skills to maximum potential	Engage client in functional tasks requiring graded challenges to shifting weight in all planes of motion while standing, bending, and reaching
	Restore functional skills in somatosensory processing to maximum potential	To improve tactile processing in hemiparetic limb: Challenge client to reach with affected hand (and vision occluded) for specified objects embedded in container filled with rice To improve vestibular processing: Present functional tasks requiring client to maintain balance during graded challenges to base of support (either sitting or standing)
	Restore functional skills in cognitive processing, planning, and performance to maximum potential	Using multicontext treatment approach, identify deficits in figure–ground discrimination and provide client with practice ignoring irrelevant details in graded tasks, such as finding a route on a map or identifying specific items on a cluttered shelf
	Restore functional social interaction skills to maximum potential	Identify social challenges client is currently experiencing, present role-playing situations (e.g., calling friend on telephone or making restaurant reservations and requesting information about accessibility), followed by client self-analysis and therapist feedback

Intervention to Modify Activity Demands and the Contexts in Which Activities Are Performed

Even with appropriate medical care and excellent rehabilitation services, many stroke survivors may fail to achieve full recovery of motor, cognitive, or perceptual skills. In addition, stroke-related fatigue may further limit their ability to perform daily activities. Participation and quality of life can be enhanced considerably through the use of strategies and equipment designed to compensate for residual impairments. Although each person deserves the opportunity to regain his or her full capacity for mobility and intellectual function, so too does each person deserve the opportunity to return to valued life activities with dignity, safety, and independence. Occupational therapists and occupational therapy assistants are experts at modifying tasks and environmental contexts to support clients' desired activity engagement within the constraints of motor, cognitive, or perceptual limitations.

During the acute stage of stroke recovery, the focus is on adapting routine self-care activities. Early rehabilitation goals include feeding oneself independently and safely, getting dressed, bathing, and performing daily grooming tasks. Although techniques are available for achieving these activities while seated and solely with the use of one arm, the skillful occupational therapist structures self-care activity performance to provide therapeutic challenges to each person's emerging balance and motor skills. Accordingly, compensatory techniques are individualized to match each person's residual skills, desire for challenge, and preferred methods of task performance.

During the rehabilitation stage, stroke survivors refine their skills in self-care activities and instrumental activities of daily living to facilitate their discharge back home. Home-based occupational therapy is critical to ensure that stroke survivors generalize newly learned skills to the environments in which they will perform the activities. Outpatient therapy provides clients with the opportunity to practice new skills at home and to consult with the occupational therapist when current strategies need modification.

During the rehabilitation stage, occupational therapists challenge stroke survivors to identify activities that are important to them within the repertoire of participation in family, community, and work roles. For many clients, however, hope for complete recovery may compete with a willingness to acknowledge the need to continue life's valued activities in ways that compensate for residual impairments. In addition, many stroke survivors are unable to predict which future activities will require adaptations for successful engagement. For example, a person might prepare for the activity demands of returning to a familiar job or routine social activity, but life continually brings new sets of challenges to all people, including active stroke survivors.

In the stage of continuing adjustment, people are faced with the everyday challenges of resuming their lives. Occupational therapy intervention to assist in problem solving for activity modification is particularly critical at this phase. Research evidence supporting the effectiveness of this type of intervention is particularly strong (Walker et al., 2004; Widen-Holmqvist et al., 1993) and is discussed in the Evidence-Based Practice section of this Guideline. Yet many stroke survivors are unable to access occupational therapy services after the rehabilitation phase. If society truly expects that stroke survivors will continue to lead active, dynamic lives, it needs to provide them with short-term interventions as necessary so they may adapt to new life demands.

For example, the birth of a first grandchild brings new joys as well as physical and cognitive challenges. A family vacation, a change in work responsibilities, a desire to access new consumer-oriented technology such as computers or entertainment programs, and the development of a new leisure pursuit all bring continued challenges for activity or environmental modifications. Two or three well-timed visits with an occupational therapist can assist the person in determining appropriate adaptive equipment, adapted strategies, and environmental modifications to enhance efficiency and safety in performance of new tasks.

The Evidence-Based Practice section of this Guideline provides evidence to support the effectiveness of occupational therapy interventions to modify activity demands and the contexts in which activities are performed to support safe, independent performance of valued activities within the constraints of motor, cognitive, or perceptual limitations.

For examples of interventions to modify activity demands, contexts, and performance patterns, see Table 5.

Environmental modifications. Environmental modifications for safety and independence depend on each client's ambulation status and capacity to use the paretic arm. For stroke survivors who are dependent on wheelchair use for mobility, occupational therapists assess the home and workplace according to national standards for wheelchair accessibility (American National Standards Institute, 2003). They make recommendations regarding ways to provide sufficient space in a driveway or garage to allow safe transfer from car to wheelchair and determine architecturally appropriate strategies to provide wheelchair accessibility at entrances, doorways, hallways, bathrooms, and rooms. Wheelchair accessibility includes sufficient space for entering; turning; and accessing switches, outlets, closets, and appliances.

Most stroke survivors who return to community living have some ability to walk. Functional ambulation, even if only for short distances, makes a significant difference in a person's ability to live safely and

Table 5. Examples of Interventions to Modify Activity Demands, Contexts, and Performance Patterns

Focus of Intervention	Desired Result	Sample Strategy
Context and environment	Modify home environment to promote safety and independence within constraints of residual deficits in performance skills	Recommend stair glide for client living in two-story home with bedrooms on second floor Recommend design layouts for home modifications to kitchen or bathroom for client who uses wheelchair
Activity demands	Modify procedures for performing valued daily activities to provide realistic challenges for using emerging motor, cognitive, or perceptual skills or to promote use of reemerging abilities	Instruct client to slide toothbrush into fisted paretic hand and brush teeth using that arm Teach client to use available lateral pinch in paretic hand to assist in donning socks
	Modify procedures for performing valued daily activities to compensate for limitations in motor, cognitive, or perceptual skills	Provide and teach client to safely use one-handed cutting board Provide and teach client to safely use rocker knife Teach client to put on shirt using modified strategy and provide client with opportunities to practice
Performance patterns	Modify daily routines to continue engaging in active lifestyle in spite of limitations in energy or motor skills	Teach client to prepare daily schedule that calls for healthy balance of activity, rest, and exercise
	Modify daily routines to maintain participation in community activities in spite of motor, cognitive, or perceptual limitations	Encourage client to use accessible transportation systems provided by community and to schedule activities according to transportation schedules

independently without the need for extensive environmental modifications. For ambulatory clients, the occupational therapist recommends modifications for stairways, helps families reorganize passage areas for unimpeded walking, and prescribes essential modifications to ensure bathroom safety. Stairway solutions may be as simple as the addition of an extra set of handrails to be used with the unaffected arm when ascending and descending the stairs. In the case of an ambulatory stroke survivor who is unable to navigate a flight of stairs, a stair glide may enable the person to maintain a bedroom safely on the second floor of the home. Bathroom modifications such as a raised toilet seat; 3-in-1 commode; tub seat; handheld shower nozzle; and safety bars for the tub, near the toilet, and at other strategic locations are critical safety interventions for stroke survivors whose balance or standing endurance is impaired.

Adaptive equipment. Adaptive equipment enables stroke survivors to perform self-care, homemaking, work, and leisure activities with varying levels of skilled motor function. Equipment selection is highly individualized and is based on the constellation of factors assessed in the occupational therapy evaluation. Some examples of widely used equipment to facilitate one-handed activity performance are a rocker knife for one-handed cutting, nonslip pads to place under plates, holders for books or playing cards, stabilizing devices for activities that traditionally require two-handed performance (e.g., cutting vegetables, cleaning dentures), and keyboards adapted for one-handed computer use. Adaptive equipment needs for driving depend on whether the left or the right limb has been affected by stroke. Most stroke survivors will benefit from a driving evaluation by a specially trained occupational therapist. Recommendations may include appropriate adaptive equipment such as a spinner knob for one-handed control of the steering wheel to enable the stroke survivor to safely return to driving. People with right hemiparesis will need adaptations allowing the left foot to control the brake and accelerator (Stav, Hunt, & Arbesman, 2006).

Intervention to Promote a Healthy and Satisfying Lifestyle

Occupational therapy practitioners help stroke survivors establish performance patterns that support adherence to medication routine, appropriate diet, appropriate levels of physical activity, and satisfying levels of engagement in social relationships and activities. Beyond developing the capacities for activity performance, stroke survivors need to establish daily routines that support their physical and emotional well-being. Unfortunately, large numbers of stroke survivors living at home report a lack of meaningful activity in their lives (Clarke, Marshall, Black, & Colantonio, 2002; Mayo et al., 2002). Engagement in activity to support participation and health is the ultimate goal of occupational therapy intervention. Artful use of the occupational profile enables an occupational therapist to target all aspects of a person's activity performance and time allocation that contribute to a healthy and satisfying lifestyle. In addition, occupational therapy intervention in every stage of stroke recovery must emphasize continued attention to the prevention of secondary impairments described earlier in this Guideline. Because stroke affects each person differently, and the context of each person's life significantly influences activity performance, each stroke survivor requires an individualized approach to promote a healthy and satisfying lifestyle.

For examples of interventions to promote a healthy lifestyle, see Table 6.

Intervention to Maintain Performance and Health

Education of clients, family, and caregivers is an important aspect of occupational therapy intervention designed to maintain performance and health after services have ended. In addition, occupational therapists develop and supervise performance of routine exercise programs designed to prevent the development of secondary impairments. Occupational therapy interventions that modify tasks and environments seek an optimal balance between safety, efficiency, and challenge to remaining skills. The presence of appropriate challenges is essential to maintaining performance capacities. Finally, occupational therapy interventions to establish active, healthy daily routines contribute further to maintaining the performance capacities of each stroke survivor and preventing an avoidable decline toward inactivity, loss of social roles, and emotional depression.

For examples of interventions to maintain performance and health, see Table 7.

Intervention Review

Intervention review is a continuous process of reevaluating and reviewing the intervention plan, the effectiveness of its delivery and the progress toward targeted outcomes (AOTA, 2008b). Reevaluation nor-

mally substantiates progress toward goal attainment, indicates any change in functional status, and directs modifications to the intervention plan, if necessary (Moyers & Dale, 2007).

Outcome Monitoring

Occupational therapists regularly monitor the results of their intervention by readministering standardized and nonstandardized assessments used in evaluation (see Table 1). This reassessment determines the need to continue or modify the intervention plan or to discontinue intervention and refer the client to other agencies or professionals. In addition, at the acute and rehabilitation stages of stroke recovery, results of occupational therapy outcomes assessment are used in determining discharge plans.

Table 6. Examples of Interventions to Promote a Healthy Lifestyle

Focus of Intervention	Desired Result	Sample Strategy
Performance patterns	Promote healthy and satisfying lifestyle that includes adherence to medication routines, appropriate diet, appropriate levels of physical activity, and satisfying levels of engagement in social relationships and activities	Engage client in individualized review of current time use, followed by active planning for realistic change Provide structured, individualized assignments for managing time and energy to be completed between therapy sessions (e.g., go to local mall and invite friend to visit)
Performance skills	Promote use of paretic arm in functional situations to maximum potential	Teach client to use Motor Activity Log (Taub et al, 1993) to set goals for use of paretic arm in specified activities and to self-monitor goal achievement

Table 7. Examples of Interventions to Maintain Performance and Health

Focus of Intervention	Desired Result	Sample Strategy
Client factors	Maintain muscle length, joint range of motion, and postural alignment	Teach client and caregivers to perform daily routine of individualized stretching and optimal postural alignment while in bed, sitting, and standing
Performance skills	Maintain improvements in balance; use of paretic limbs; and cognitive, perceptual, and emotional coping skills	Modify daily activities to provide ongoing appropriate challenges to current skills*

* Challenges are based on ongoing monitoring and assessment of residual and emerging performance skills, mechanical constraints, and performance patterns.

Occupational therapy practitioners document outcomes just as they document evaluation findings and interventions (AOTA, 2008a). They complete this documentation within the time frames, formats, and standards established by practice settings, agencies, external accreditation programs, and payers (AOTA, 2005).

In addition to monitoring outcomes of individuals, occupational therapists use aggregate data from outcomes assessments to evaluate the effectiveness of specific interventions. This use of standardized outcomes data is critical for program development and the establishment of a research foundation for evidence-based practice.

Discontinuation, Discharge Planning, and Follow-up

Ideally, planning for discharge begins at the time a stroke survivor starts to participate in an occupational therapy treatment program.

Early planning ensures that treatment will provide the best preparation for the person's future success after services are discontinued. In many situations, clients are discharged from occupational therapy services at a particular site before all the treatment goals have been met. In these cases, it is important to document which outcomes have not yet been achieved and to recommend occupational therapy and other professional services that are provided through other venues. For example, when a stroke survivor is discharged home from a rehabilitation facility, home-based or outpatient occupational therapy services usually are indicated. When home-based services must be terminated for reimbursement reasons, clients need access to potential resources for private-pay or grant-funded interventions. In the absence of resources for continued occupational therapy intervention, therapists are obligated to provide clients and caregivers with clear, written instructions for ongoing home management and information about community agencies providing continuing support or activity programs.

Occupational therapy services may be indicated at several points throughout the life of a stroke survivor. There is significant research evidence that occupational therapy services can promote independence, health, and quality of life (Legg, Drummond, & Langhorne, 2006). The current health care system needs to develop improved mechanisms to ensure that stroke survivors can access short-term occupational therapy services to meet their evolving needs, as determined by changes in physical status, environment, and life roles.

■ ■ ■

Evidence-Based Practice

One of the greatest challenges facing health care systems, service providers, public educators, and policymakers is to ensure that scarce resources are used efficiently. This has influenced a growing interest in outcomes research and evidenced-based medicine over the past three decades.

In response to demands of the cost-oriented health care system in which occupational therapy practice often is embedded, occupational therapists and occupational therapy assistants are routinely asked to justify the value of the services they provide on the basis of scientific evidence. The scientific literature provides an important source of legitimacy and authority for demonstrating the value of health care and education services. Thus, occupational therapists and other health care professionals increasingly are called on to use the literature to demonstrate the value of the interventions and instruction they provide to clients and students.

After due consideration, there is now international consensus in the occupational therapy profession about the appropriateness of establishing standards based on a review of the literature on the effectiveness of occupational therapy interventions (Law & Baum, 1998; Taylor & Savin-Baden, 2001; Tickle-Degnen, 1999, 2000; Tickle-Degnen, Baker, & Murphy, 2001).

Concurrent with the movement toward increased accountability and restraint in health care spending, there has been an internal demand for the development of standards for the practice of occupational therapy. Both trends have led to shifts in occupational therapy clinical decision making toward the use of professional judgment and knowledge of individual client characteristics and preferences in tandem with evidence from scientific literature (Sackett, Rosenberg, Muir Gray, Haynes, & Richardson, 1996). That is, occupational therapy practice has expanded to unite clinical reasoning with evidence from scientific literature and client characteristics and preferences.

To assist therapists in gaining access to findings from scientific literature, AOTA has sponsored a series of evidence-based literature reviews of the effectiveness of occupational therapy interventions for a variety of health and developmental conditions. This Guideline incorporates the findings from the work related to occupational therapy and stroke.

What Is an Evidence-Based Practice Perspective?

According to Law and Baum (1998), evidence-based occupational therapy practice "uses research evidence together with clinical knowledge and reasoning to make decisions about interventions that are effective for a specific client" (p. 131). An evidence-based perspective is based on the assumption that the strength of scientific evidence can be judged according to a hierarchy of research designs and an assessment of the quality of the research. AOTA uses a grading system based on standards from evidence-based medicine. This system standardizes and ranks the value of scientific evidence for biomedical practice using the grading criteria in Table 8. The highest levels of evidence are produced by studies that are systematic reviews of the literature, meta-analyses, and randomized controlled trials. In randomized controlled trials, the outcomes of an intervention group are compared with the outcomes of a control group, and participation in either group is determined randomly. The evidence-based literature reviews presented here include Level I studies, which are randomized controlled trials, systematic reviews, or meta-analyses; Level II studies, in which assignment to a treatment or a control group is not randomized (cohort studies); Level III studies, which use one-group pretest–posttest or before–after designs; Level IV studies, which are single-case experimental

Table 8. Levels of Evidence for Occupational Therapy Outcomes Research

Levels of Evidence	Definitions
Level I	Systematic reviews, meta-analyses, randomized controlled trials
Level II	Two groups, nonrandomized studies (e.g., cohort, case-control)
Level III	One group, nonrandomized (e.g., before and after, pretest and posttest)
Level IV	Descriptive studies that include analysis of outcomes (e.g., single-subject design, case series)
Level V	Case reports and expert opinion that include narrative literature reviews and consensus statements

Adapted from "Evidence-based medicine: What it is and what it isn't," by D. L. Sackett, W. M. Rosenberg, J. A. Muir Gray, R. B. Haynes, & W. S. Richardson, 1996, *British Medical Journal, 312*, pp. 71–72.

designs, sometimes reported over several participants; and Level V studies, which reflect expert opinion, including narrative literature reviews and consensus statements.

Best Practices in Intervention With Stroke Survivors: Results of the Evidence-Based Literature Review

This Guideline is based on two systematic reviews:
1. An evidence-based literature review conducted in the early 2000s, addressing the effectiveness of occupational therapy with people who had experienced a stroke
2. A broad-based review conducted in 2003, seeking basic scientific information to develop this Guideline and data on the effectiveness of any therapy in reducing impairment in people who had experienced a stroke.

Methodology for the First Review

The authors of the first review were Catherine A. Trombly Latham, ScD, OTR/L, FAOTA, and Hui-ing Ma, ScD, OTR/L. They searched the literature published from 1980 to 2000, focusing on therapeutic goals: restoration of roles, tasks, and activities and remediation of impaired bodily functions.

Specific inclusion criteria were as follows:
- The study was published in a peer-reviewed journal from 1980 to 2000, was included in a systematic review published from 1980 to 2000, or was a thesis or dissertation completed from 1980 to 2000 in the English language. The team excluded reports published before 1980 "because knowledge of motor behavior and recovery after central nervous system damage that affect therapeutic procedures as well as the philosophy of occupational therapy practice were different 20 years ago and [might] not be currently applicable" (Trombly & Ma, 2002, p. 251).
- The study measured the effect of occupational therapy treatment of people who had experienced a stroke.
- The intervention described in each study was designated as occupational therapy or administered by an occupational therapist, or the article was written by an occupational therapist.

Trombly and Ma first identified key words for the search: *occupational therapy AND stroke OR cerebrovascular accident (CVA), cerebrovascular disorders, hemiplegia, hemiparesis,* or *hemiplegics.* Then they searched the literature. They began with a manual search of the following journals:
- *American Journal of Occupational Therapy*
- *British Journal of Occupational Therapy*

- *Canadian Journal of Occupational Therapy*
- *Occupational Therapy in Health Care*
- *Occupational Therapy Journal of Research*
- *Physical and Occupational Therapy in Geriatrics.*

Next, they searched the following electronic databases:

- Cumulative Index to Nursing and Allied Health Literature (1981–2000)
- Dissertation Abstracts (1980–2000)
- Excerpta Medica, Volume 19: Rehabilitation and Physical Medicine (1980–2000)
- Index Medicus (1980–1983)
- MEDLINE (1984–2000)
- PsychLit (1980–2000)
- Social Science Citation Index (1988–2000).

They also examined the reference sections of relevant articles for additional studies. They continued tracking citations until they found no new studies.

The reviewers found 150 articles, which they then evaluated for quality (scientific rigor and lack of bias) and levels of evidence. Thirty-six articles met their criteria and were included in the review.

Fifteen of the 36 articles addressed restoration. (Eight of the 15 also addressed remediation.) The reviewers classified 10 of the 15 as Level I studies, 2 as Level II studies, and 3 as Level III studies.

All 15 studies were conducted in a natural setting (in the participants' homes or in clinics). They included an initial total of 984 participants, 895 (91%) of whom completed the studies. Of these, 411 had a lesion on the left side of the brain, and 425 had one on the right side. Two studies did not report the location of the lesion. Participants in 4 studies were in the chronic stage (12 months or more since the stroke), when little spontaneous recovery is expected (Gresham et al., 1995; Wade, 1992). Participants in 10 studies were in the acute stage (6 months or less since the stroke, when spontaneous recovery is considered to

be occurring).[2] Participants in one study were of mixed chronicity. Twenty-nine of the 36 studies included in the initial review addressed remediation. The reviewers classified 17 of these as Level I studies, 9 as Level II studies, 2 as Level III studies, and 1 as a Level IV study.

Seventeen (59%) studies were applied research on therapy offered in clinical or home settings, and 12 (41%) were reports of experimental treatment or research designed to understand the nature of the clients' responses to treatment applied under laboratory conditions. The 29 studies included an initial total of 832 participants (37 healthy people and 795 stroke survivors), 797 of whom completed the studies. Three hundred seventeen participants had a lesion on the left side of the brain, and 328 on the right. Four studies did not report the location of the lesion. Twelve of the studies included participants who had sustained their strokes at least 1 year earlier. The remaining 12 studies included participants whose stroke had occurred within the past 7 months.

The results of the review were published in two parts, corresponding with the two focuses: restoration (Trombly & Ma, 2002) and remediation (Ma & Trombly, 2002).

Methodology for the Second Review

The reviewer for the second review was Dr. Trombly Latham. This review included 11 questions and focused on two topics areas identified by an expert panel: the neurophysiological basis of poststroke brain reorganization and interventions for poststroke recovery in impairments, activities, and participation. This Guideline incorporates some of the findings from this review. Inclusion criteria varied between the two topics.

The expert group designed the first six questions to target information from the basic sciences needed to write this Guideline. The criteria were as follows:

---

[2]In the stroke literature, spontaneous recovery is considered negligible after 12 months but ongoing until then, with the greatest changes expected up to 6 months. In research, the participants whose strokes occurred at least 12 months earlier act as controls for spontaneous recovery as an alternative explanation of the outcome.

- The study or the review was published in a peer-reviewed journal in the English language from 1997–2002.[3]
- The article specifically addressed the particular question posed and included laboratory animal studies and human studies. The subjects included rats and monkeys as well as humans.

The expert group designed the final five questions around the effectiveness of interventions. The focus of the first intervention question was to evaluate the effectiveness of occupational therapy interventions for remediating impairments or restoring activities and participation after stroke. The criteria were the same as those for the 2002 Trombly and Ma review, except that the search period was from 2000–2002 to cover the time since the 2002 review was completed. Three focused questions addressed the effectiveness of therapeutic interventions to address psychological, social, and perceptual impairments and promote participation. An additional focused question targeted the effectiveness of constraint-induced therapy to improve behavioral outcomes following stroke.

The criteria for this group of focused questions included articles both within and related to the occupational therapy literature:

- The study or the review was published in a peer-reviewed journal in the English language from 1997–2002.
- The study measured the effect of interventions within the scope of occupational therapy practice on people who had experienced a stroke.

Key words for the search were *stroke AND recovery, functional MRI AND brain reorganization, task-specificity AND recovery, environment AND recovery AND stroke, context AND motor behavior AND stroke, context AND motor behavior, stroke AND hemorrhage AND infarct OR embolism AND outcome, task demand AND recovery, practice AND recovery AND brain, stroke AND recovery AND intensity, learning AND stroke, stroke AND recovery AND unilateral neglect, brain reorganization AND stroke, stroke AND recovery AND cognition, stroke AND recovery AND adaptation, stroke AND recovery AND apraxia, occupational therapy AND stroke (2000–2002), forced use therapy AND stroke,* and *constraint-induced therapy.* The reviewer also searched for articles by recognized experts in neuroplasticity: M. Hallett, B. Kopp, J. Liepert, and R. J. Nudo.

The reviewer searched the following resources:

- Electronic databases (MEDLINE, PsycINFO, Web of Science [Science Citation Index and Social Science Citation Index]).
- Consolidated information sources (e.g., evidence-based medicine reviews such as the Cochrane Database of Systematic Reviews; the Cochrane Controlled Trials Register; DARE—the Database of Abstracts of Reviews of Effectiveness, published by the British National Health Service; and the National Guidelines Clearinghouse, part of the Agency for Health Research and Quality, U.S. National Institutes of Health). The entries in these sources are peer reviewed, but they are not journal articles. The sources provide a system for clinicians and scientists to conduct evidence-based reviews of selected clinical questions and topics (Hayes & McGrath, 1998).

The reviewer also manually searched journals not indexed in the preceding databases (e.g., *Journal of Motor Behavior* and *Motor Control*).

Finally, the reviewer examined the reference sections of relevant articles for classic articles.

The reviewer selected 386 abstracts as possibly pertinent to the questions. On closer examination, she selected 122 for retrieval. She evaluated them for specificity to the questions and, if they reported a study, for quality (scientific rigor and lack of bias)

---

[3]The original plan was to cover 1992–2002 (starting from when the previous literature search on stroke had ended) but to emphasize the last 5 years (1997–2002). The review included some pre-1992 classic articles that addressed the questions. After the literature search, because of the number of articles that emerged, the scope was reduced to 1997–2002, except for the pre-1992 classics and a few studies from 1992–1997 that were occupational therapy interventions and directly addressed the questions.

and levels of evidence. She included 106 articles in her review, only 58 (54.7%) of which were research studies.

The results of this review addressing the 11 focused questions can be found in the Evidence-Based Practice section of the member area of the AOTA Web site.

Since 2003, additional articles were added (including systematic reviews and randomized controlled trials from within and related to the occupational therapy literature) to provide more recent information on specific topics (e.g., neuroplasticity, constraint-induced movement therapy, robotics) with particular relevance to occupational therapy and stroke. The following review of the evidence consists of descriptions of selected studies identified in the evidence-based literature review, information about their strengths and weaknesses based on the study design and methodology, and presentations of their findings relevant to the effect of occupational therapy treatment of stroke survivors. All studies identified by the reviews and described in this section are summarized in the evidence tables in Appendix B. Readers are encouraged to read the full articles for more details.

Evidence for the Efficacy of Occupational Therapy Interventions With Stroke Survivors

An evidence-based review of the literature using methods and classifications described on pages 39–40 of this document provides the following support for occupational therapy intervention with stroke survivors:

- Neural plasticity is possible after mammalian brain lesions and is positively influenced by specific types of task-based environmental challenges.
- Occupational therapy interventions are effective in remediating motor and process skills after stroke. These skill improvements are related to improvements in functional activities.
- Occupational therapy effectively improves the capacity of stroke survivors to perform tasks,

activities, and roles independently. These improvements are often associated with improvements in self-perceived quality of life.

Neural Plasticity and Task-Based Environmental Challenges

Plasticity, the brain's capacity to dynamically reorganize, has been demonstrated systematically in studies of skill learning in healthy adults, in studies examining recovery after experimental lesions to mammalian brains, and in studies of human stroke survivors who demonstrate behavioral recovery. Research findings overwhelmingly support the importance of activity-based environmental challenges and repetitive practice opportunities in facilitating this neural reorganization.

Studies of Skill Learning in Healthy Human Adults

Noninvasive techniques of positron emission tomography (PET scans), functional magnetic resonance imaging (fMRI), and transcranial magnetic stimulation (TMS) allow researchers to study neural activity of specific brain regions and, delineate cortical representation areas for selected observable behaviors. Numerous studies of healthy adults have established that extensive task practice and subsequent skill development is related to concomitant increases in cortical representation areas for the associated function. For example, a seminal Level II study (Sadato et al., 1998) used PET imaging to measure regional cerebral blood flow while two groups of subjects performed a variety of tactile tasks with the right index finger. Experimental group participants were 8 experienced Braille readers who had been blind for most of their lives. Ten sighted subjects without Braille experience served as controls. PET scans revealed distinctly different cortical activation patterns in the two groups as subjects performed the same tasks. As expected, when sighted subjects performed tactile discrimination tasks, the most significant cortical activation was in the secondary somatosensory area (typically associated with tactile processing). In the blind Braille readers, however, occipital regions (typically associated with visual processing) were activated during the same, tactile-oriented activities. This study set a foundation for the current understanding that with extensive practice reading Braille, the neural networks for tactile processing are rerouted to cortical regions originally reserved for visual discrimination.

A more recent Level II study (Saito, Okada, Honda, Yonekura, & Sadato, 2006) used *f* MRI to compare cortical activation between two groups of normally sighted adults. Experimental group participants were expert players of Mah-jong, a game involving flat plastic tiles with various marks carved on one side. These expert players had developed an ability to identify the carved patterns by touch, thus improving their tactile discrimination abilities to such extraordinary levels that they were able to visualize the patterns through touch. Control group participants had no previous experience playing Mah-jong. Participants were tested on two assessments of tactile discrimination, one involving Mah-jong tiles and one involving Braille characters, with which both groups were unfamiliar. As expected, when compared with the control group, Mah-jong experts demonstrated significantly greater accuracy on the Mah-jong task but comparable performance on the Braille task. When compared with the *f* MRI results for the control group, activation of the visual cortex was significantly greater for the expert group on both tasks. This result indicates cross-modal neural plasticity produced by the effects of long-term training with the Mah-jong tiles.

Animal Lesion Studies

Studies of mammals with experimentally induced cortical lesions consistently find that after an acute critical period of approximately 1 week in which overuse is detrimental to recovery (Humm, Kozlowski, James Gotts, & Schallert, 1998), disuse of an impaired forelimb has a negative impact upon behavioral recovery and cortical representation of the immobilized limb (Friel, Heddings, & Nudo, 2000; Leasure & Schallert, 2004). Conversely, factors promoting purposeful use of impaired forelimbs, such as enriched environments (Johansson, 1996, 2003) and task training (Biernaskie & Corbett, 2001; Brown, Bjelke, & Fuxe, 2004; Jones, Chu, Grande, & Gregory, 1999), have signifi-

cant positive effects on behavioral recovery and cortical reorganization.

For example, in a Level II study, Friel, Heddings, and Nudo (2000) induced lesions in the hand representation area of the primary motor cortex of squirrel monkeys, then tested the monkeys under three conditions: (1) no intervention, (2) restraint of the unaffected arm and hand with no training, and (3) restraint of the unaffected arm and hand with training. One month after the lesion, the restraint-with-training group showed significantly greater spared hand area (area not damaged by the lesion) than either of the other groups. Indeed, the restraint-with-training group had increased its spared hand area by 9%, whereas the other two groups had lost more than 50% of their spared hand areas. Also, the restraint-with-training group showed significantly greater spared digit area than the no-intervention group and tended to show greater spared digit area than the restraint-without-training group. The researchers concluded that repetitive use of the impaired hand is necessary for sparing the associated region in the primary motor cortex.

In a Level I study with multiple treatment and control groups, Leasure and Schallert (2004) induced unilateral lesions or sham operations in the forelimb representation area of the sensorimotor cortex of rats. They then assigned the rats to groups involving immobilization (disuse) of the paretic forelimb through plaster casting at varying points in time after the lesion and for varying durations, ranging from 7 days to 14 days. Their most critical finding was that lesioned rats in the "early disuse group" showed significantly slower recovery of bilateral limb use as compared to all other rats in the study. In addition, they found that early disuse extended the period in which these animals were vulnerable to overuse atrophy of remaining brain tissue. The implications are that notwithstanding earlier findings of brain atrophy associated with limb overuse too soon after an experimentally induced brain lesion, complete disuse during this critical period has significantly greater functional consequences.

Several studies provide support for the value of enriched environments and task training to behavioral recovery and cortical reorganization in mammals with experimentally induced brain lesions. In a Level II nonrandomized controlled trial, Johansson (1996) tested 15 rats that had undergone focal brain ischemia. The focus of the research was to determine whether transferring some of the rats to an enriched environment after housing all of them in standard cages for 2 weeks following surgery would improve outcomes. The rats in the enriched environment significantly improved their prehensile traction, limb placement, and performance on a rotating pole.

Other studies have yielded similar results with task training. In a Level II nonrandomized controlled trial, Biernaskie and Corbett (2001) compared rats housed in enriched conditions that included areas for exploration, variety in the cage, and daily rehabilitative training with rats without those enriched conditions. Rats in the enriched conditions had significantly better performance on reaching and beam-walking tasks. Postmortem examination revealed statistically significant differences between the two groups in dendritic reorganization within the intact hemisphere. The researchers concluded that the combination of an enriched environment and task-oriented motor challenges promoted neural plasticity and functional improvements in motor function.

Brown, Bjelke, and Fuxe (2004), in a Level I randomized controlled trial, trained rats to walk beams, induced lesions on them, then tested their beam walking for 10 days under various experimental conditions: 2 hours of additional training, a dose of amphetamine, limited trials, and combinations of these conditions. Training produced the most motor recovery, amphetamine treatment delayed it, and limited experience had a negative effect.

In a Level I randomized controlled trial, Jones et al. (1999) induced lesions in the forelimb representation area of the sensorimotor cortex of rats and then trained them in an acrobatic task. Earlier studies had shown such lesions and acrobatic training independently to increase synapse-to-neuron ratios in the motor cortex opposite the site of the lesion. In this study, combining the two interventions resulted in enhanced synapse-to-neuron ratios in the same area. They concluded that

behavioral therapy can facilitate adaptive neural plasticity.

Some neuroscientists who study motor learning in animals are deliberate in differentiating task-based practice from repetitive movement. In a Level I randomized controlled trial, Plautz, Milliken, and Nudo (2000) studied the effects of repetitive use without learning in squirrel monkeys who received a surgically imposed infarction of the primary motor area of the cortex. The task required the monkeys to retrieve a food pellet from a well that was wide enough to accommodate their whole hand. This was an automatic response for the monkeys and did not require them to learn a new motor task. The researchers evaluated whether repetitive motor activity was sufficient to result in representational plasticity in cortical motor maps or whether learning was needed. The data confirmed that after 12,000 trials, the monkeys had not learned any new motor skills in the task activity. Examination of the cortical motor maps of the simple repetitive activity revealed no systematic task-related changes in representations. The researchers compared these results with those of an earlier Level I randomized controlled trial (Nudo, Milliken, Jenkins, & Merzenich, 1996). The monkeys in the 1996 study had performed a similar task but with a well of smaller width, which required the monkeys to learn a new motor skill. In the study where the monkeys were required to learn a new motor skill, the researchers found both behavioral changes and motor cortex reorganization. Plautz and colleagues concluded that the development of learned skills through attempts to meet environmental challenges serves as the impetus for an injured central nervous system to reorganize itself.

Accordingly, researchers are careful to rearrange enriched environments frequently so that the recovering animals are presented with varying opportunities for exploration (e.g., Biernaskie & Corbett, 2001). In addition, they design the training tasks to be inherently motivating for the animals (e.g., Biernaskie & Corbett, 2001; Jones et al., 1999). Occupational therapy interventions to restore motor, cognitive, and perceptual skills in human stroke survivors are entirely compatible with this principle, which routinely informs the design of neuroplasticity research with animals. When working with human stroke survivors, occupational therapists design task-based environmental challenges. They individualize the opportunities for practice to ensure that the opportunities are both meaningful to the client and represent an appropriate level of difficulty.

Studies of Human Stroke Survivors

Level V reviews of neuroimaging studies of human stroke survivors (Dancause, 2006; Rossini et al., 2007) conclude that recovery of motor function after brain injury is associated with recruitment of brain regions not typically activated for a specific behavior. In a descriptive study, Cramer et al. (1997) compared fMRI findings during index-finger tapping by 10 patients who had recovered hand movements after stroke and by 9 healthy people who acted as controls. They found that motor recovery after stroke is accompanied by increased activity in the unaffected sensorimotor cortex as well as the premotor cortex and the supplementary motor area in the affected hemisphere.

In another descriptive study, Thickbroom, Byrnes, Archer, and Mastaglia (2004) investigated the relationship between reorganization of the motor cortex and degree of motor function following a subcortical stroke. They performed TMS mapping of long-term stroke survivors with and without extensive motor recovery. They found that the degree of cortical reorganization is related to improvements in arm motor function and grip strength.

Functional recovery depends on some degree of fiber sparing. Most studies to date have examined motor function in the hand, and research has identified corticospinal tract integrity as being critical to functional recovery. For example, in a descriptive study, Binkofski et al. (1996) examined whether lesional and remote depressions of regional cerebral glucose metabolism (rCMRGlu) and the severity of corticospinal (pyramidal) tract involvement were related to motor recovery in the early chronic stage after hemiparetic stroke. They found that motor recovery was related both to the extent of pyramidal tract involvement and to remote rCMRGlu depression in the thalamus occurring on the same side as the stroke lesion.

Foltys et al. (2003) studied 10 stroke survivors who demonstrated rapid and extensive motor recovery. They compared fMRI and TMS findings when these subjects used their recovered hand, as compared with the nonaffected hand, to perform simple and complex hand tasks. (The simple task was repeated mass finger flexion and release. The complex task was repeated thumb opposition to subsequent fingers.) Like other studies that provide support for functional cortical reorganization, this study found statistically significant increases in activation of the contralateral supplementary motor area, the contralateral cerebellum, and the ipsilateral primary motor area (M1) when subjects used their recovered hand as compared to their nonaffected hand. In addition, though, the finding of similar activation from M1 in both the affected and nonaffected hemispheres suggests that fiber sparing in the affected primary motor cortex is a necessary requirement for rapid motor recovery.

The caveat of these descriptive studies—that functional recovery depends on some degree of fiber sparing—has implications for the understanding of occupational therapy interventions. The research evidence supporting mechanisms of brain plasticity after stroke is clearly a source of optimism. However, clients and therapists must acknowledge that only rehabilitation interventions can help stroke survivors reach their maximum potential for recovery. This potential, which cannot be assessed in typical clinical situations, depends on physiological and anatomical factors.

In the presence of sufficient remaining function in associated neuronal pathways, neural plasticity (or cortical reorganization) seems to be the primary process for recovery of function after stroke. Neuroscience studies consistently find that task-based environmental challenges are the most effective mechanism for promoting this cortical reorganization. These findings have led to the development and testing of constraint-induced movement therapy (CIMT), an increasingly validated intervention for stroke survivors who meet motor criteria of active wrist and finger extension as well as high-level balance and cognitive skills. Several studies have used neuroimaging techniques to provide evidence of changes in neural organization following CIMT. In these studies (Liepert, 2006 [Level III]; Liepert et al. 2000 [Level III]; Liepert, Hamzei, & Weiller, 2004 [Level III]; Wittenberg et al., 2003 [Level I]), the researchers consistently challenged participants who exhibited some anatomical sparing to motor pathways to use their paretic arm and hand for functional tasks through constraint of the unaffected upper limb. Significant improvements in functional arm use were accompanied by changes in cortical organization.

Liepert and colleagues (2000), in a Level III study with a pretest–posttest design, used TMS to assess the plasticity brought about by CIMT. Following treatment, the size of the muscle output area in the affected hemisphere was significantly enlarged (nearly double in size), which corresponded with improved performance of the paretic limb and reported increases in use of the paretic limb during daily activities.

In a Level III study, Liepert et al. (2004) found that CIMT resulted in changes in intracortical excitability, mainly in the affected hemisphere, as measured by TMS and fMRI. In a Level I randomized controlled trial Wittenberg and colleagues (2003) compared the effects of CIMT and a less-intensive intervention on motor function and brain physiology in stroke patients. Along with significant improvement in functional performance, TMS revealed observable changes in cortical activation by patients in the experimental group. Specifically, those patients recruited larger areas of their affected hemisphere's motor cortex. No changes were evident in the patients in the control group.

In a Level III study with a before-and-after design, Liepert (2006) used TMS and functional motor tests to examine inhibitory and facilitatory neuronal circuits in the primary motor cortex of patients in the chronic phase of stroke who were participating in a 12-day program of CIMT. They also examined the mechanisms involved in therapy-associated modulations of motor excitability. One finding was that clinical spasticity, as measured by the Ashworth Test of Spasticity, is associated with a decrease in intracortical inhibition as measured by TMS. After participating in the CIMT program, the patients demonstrated clinical decreases in spasticity, which were associated with pronounced increases in intracortical inhibition.

In summary, the neuroscience literature provides extensive support for the human brain's capacity to reorganize for functional recovery after stroke. Furthermore, the research evidence indicates that provision of task-based environmental challenges may be the most effective method for facilitating this recovery. Occupational therapy's foundational tenet of providing client-centered, activity-based practice opportunities to improve targeted skills in stroke survivors is consistent with current concepts and findings by neuroscience researchers.

Intervention to Improve Motor Skills

A moderate-sized body of evidence supports the efficacy of occupational therapy intervention in improving motor skills after stroke. This evidence has been analyzed in two Level I systematic reviews in English that are specific to occupational therapy (Ma & Trombly, 2002; Steultjens et al., 2003) and in practice guidelines for rehabilitation of stroke survivors (Gresham et al., 1995; New Zealand Guidelines Group, 2003; Ottawa Panel, 2006; Scottish Intercollegiate Guidelines Network, 2002; Stroke Canada Optimization of Rehabilitation through Evidence [SCORE], 2007).

Intervention to Improve Client Factors Related to Movement

Motor skill is a person's ability to harness available movement for functional performance. In stroke survivors, improvements in motor skill are intrinsically dependent upon a person's capacity to generate movement, as well as on prevention and management of secondary motor impairments. Following a Level I systematic review of treatment interventions for the paretic upper limb of stroke survivors, Barreca, Wolf, Fasoli, and Bohannon (2003) advised therapists to determine the focus of their interventions based on each patient's current and expected degree of recovery. A specific focus on regaining upper-limb motor skill is appropriate for the select group of stroke survivors who exhibit the capacity to produce a repertoire of active movements. When working with stroke survivors who exhibit minimal motor recovery in the paretic arm, treatment should focus on maintaining comfort and passive mobility and emphasize improving skills in other areas, such as balance, gross mobility, emotional adjustment, and occupational performance.

Intervention to Manage Secondary Impairments

Some interventions geared toward reducing secondary motor impairments in stroke survivors have been supported through published research evidence. For reduction of hand edema, active movement in conjunction with elevation is more effective than elevation alone (Level I; Barreca et al., 2003). Barreca and colleagues (2003) also reported collective evidence that supports the benefits of a home exercise program that emphasizes self-range of motion of the paretic arm. In addition to the research reviewed by Barreca and colleagues, one Level I study (Nelson et al., 1996) randomly assigned 30 participants to one of two groups focused on improving passive range of motion (PROM) in forearm supination. Passive limitation in forearm supination is common in stroke survivors who present with spasticity, and affects performance of activities such as bathing and dressing. Participants in the treatment group performed the range of motion (ROM) exercise within the context of a dice game in which the person was required to rotate a handle to varying extents to release colored dice from a therapeutic device that was specially designed for this study. Nelson and colleagues labeled this treatment "occupationally embedded exercise." Participants in the control group were instructed to perform the supination ROM exercises without the context of a game. Nelson and colleagues (1996) reported that, during task performance, stroke survivors who performed occupationally embedded exercise achieved PROM for forearm supination that was statistically significantly greater than the PROM achieved by members of the control group.

For prevention and management of shoulder subluxation, Price and Pandyan's (2000) Level I systematic Cochrane Review reported that electrical stimulation applied to the posterior deltoid and supraspinatus muscles is effective in improving degree of subluxation as well as pain-free ROM for passive humeral lateral rotation. However, there is no evidence that electrical stimulation has a significant impact on the incidence or intensity of shoulder pain in stroke survivors. Barreca and colleagues (2003) reported preliminary evidence in support of shoulder strapping to manage shoulder subluxation.

There is little supporting evidence for some other interventions to manage secondary motor impairments. Despite numerous studies, two Level I systematic reviews reported that there is insufficient evidence to support the use of resting hand splints as a routine intervention in stroke rehabilitation (Lannin & Herbert, 2003; Ma & Trombly, 2002). A Level I Cochrane Systematic Review (Ada et al., 2005) concluded that there is insufficient evidence to determine whether conventional shoulder slings and wheelchair attachments prevent subluxation, decrease pain, or increase function in the paretic shoulder after stroke.

Intervention to Enhance Motor Recovery

Level I systematic reviews of research studies investigating electrical stimulation, biofeedback, and the combination of these two techniques (also called "electromyography-triggered neuromuscular stimulation") have provided evidence for their efficacy in improving patients' capacity to produce individual movements (Barreca et al., 2003; Pomeroy, King, Pollock, Baily-Hallan, & Langhorne, 2006; Woodford & Price, 2007). However, findings have been limited to short-term impact, and the understanding is that these modalities must be used in conjunction with or as immediate predecessors to task-based interventions if the goal is to improve motor skill (Page & Levine, 2006).

The research literature about neurofacilitation techniques, including Proprioceptive Neuromuscular Facilitation, the Rood Approach, and the Brunnstrom

Approach, is sparse and inconclusive. Furthermore, these interventions are based on outdated views of motor recovery and motor control (Ma & Trombly, 2002; Pollock, Baer, Pomeroy, & Langhorne, 2007; Steultjens et al., 2003). Neurodevelopmental treatment (NDT), a continually evolving approach to rehabilitation (Howle, 2002), is based loosely on the historical writings of Karel and Berta Bobath (Bobath, 1978) and is called the Bobath approach in Europe. Two Level I systematic reviews (Luke, Dodd, & Brock, 2004; Paci, 2003) did not find evidence of significantly better outcomes for NDT when compared with other treatments to improve motor function in stroke survivors. However, a more recent Level I randomized controlled study with stroke patients in the rehabilitation phase found significantly greater change scores on measures affecting balance and functional leg movement for patients who participated in 4 weeks of NDT intervention when compared with a control group who received equal doses of orthopedic treatment during that time (Wang, Chen, Chen, & Yang, 2005).

Task-Based Practice Opportunities to Improve Motor Skill

A significant and growing body of research evidence, from within occupational therapy as well as other professions, supports the effectiveness of providing task-based practice opportunities to improve motor skills in those stroke survivors who demonstrate specified levels of movement capacity.

Task-Based Practice Opportunities to Improve Lower-Limb Function and Balance

In a Level I randomized controlled trial using a counterbalanced repeated-measures design, Hsieh, Nelson, Smith, and Peterson (1996) compared the dynamic standing performances of stroke patients on two types of activity engagement (actually throwing balls and the mental practice of imagining themselves throwing balls) with a rote exercise that involved similar movements. The results of the study indicate that participants performed significantly more repetitions when either actually throwing a ball or imagining themselves throwing a ball as compared to rote exercise. In a Level II nonrandomized controlled trial, also using a counterbalanced repeated-measures design, Dolecheck and Schkade (1999) compared the effectiveness of therapeutic activities that were personally meaningful and goal directed with the effectiveness of activities that were not in improving the dynamic standing balance of stroke patients. Both studies found that dynamic standing endurance improved when persons with hemiplegia performed meaningful activities in the context of an exercise regimen to improve bending down, reaching, standing up, or using their arm while standing.

A Level I systematic review of studies using repetitive task training to improve functional ability after stroke (French et al., 2007) included randomized and quasi-randomized trials in which the intervention consisted of an active motor sequence that was performed repetitively within the context of a task with a clear functional goal. Many of the 14 studies that met the criteria for this review tested interventions associated with motor relearning approaches that have been articulated by Carr and Shepherd (1998, 2003), Winstein and Knecht (1990), and other movement scientists (Schmidt & Lee, 2005; Shumway-Cook & Woollacott, 2006). Based on the collective analysis of the aggregate data from the 14 studies included in their systematic review, French and colleagues (2007) found that task-related training, when compared to a variety of exercise-based control interventions, led to significantly greater improvements in activities of daily living, walking distance, walking speed, and functional aspects of sit-to-stand. The collective analysis of aggregate data did not yield statistically significant differences for balance outcomes. However, the review included a Level I randomized controlled trial with 20 participants who were at least 1 year poststroke that did provide support for the value of task-related training in improving seated reaching, as compared to a control treatment that provided no challenges to the participants to shift their centers of mass while sitting (Dean & Shepherd, 1997). Participants in a 2-week task-related training program aimed at increasing both the distance of reach and the level of support from the paretic leg during seated reaching performed significantly better than control participants on (1) ability to reach faster and further, (2) increased load through the affected foot, and (3) increased activation of extensor muscles in the affected leg. These gains also led to functional improvements in speed and efficiency in sit-to-stand.

Task-Based Practice Opportunities to Improve Arm and Hand Motor Skill

Effect of Object Affordances on Skilled Use of the Arm and Hand in Stroke Survivors

A series of studies using motion-analysis technology found that key kinematic variables are improved when stroke survivors use their paretic upper limb to use functional objects, as compared with when they perform similar movement sequences in the absence of task performance. These studies with stroke survivors are based on a body of knowledge derived from earlier studies in the movement science literature about object affordances, motor learning, and motor control. *Object affordances* are the immediate perceptions an object generates in its potential user as to how the object can potentially be used to accomplish something. For example, when a human adult sees a coffee mug, he or she immediately perceives its affordance as something to be picked up by the handle and brought to the mouth for drinking coffee. Motor control begins *before* actual performance begins. Humans and other animals begin to develop a motor plan with the initial perception of an object's affordances. The object's purpose, location, size, and perceived weight all play a role in generating the motor plan and ultimately influence various aspects of the movement sequence.

In a Level I randomized controlled trial using a counterbalanced repeated measures design, Wu, Trombly, Lin, and Tickle-Degnen (1998) tested the effects of object affordances on reaching performance in persons with and without hemiparesis under two conditions: enriched object affordances and impoverished object affordances. Wu and colleagues defined enriched object affordances as a situation in which the person interacts with an object whose purpose is well understood. In this study, during the enriched

affordances condition, participants reached forward to a familiar household chopping gadget and were instructed to push down the handle to chop a fresh mushroom. Wu and colleagues defined impoverished affordances as a situation in which the person has no knowledge of an object's purpose and is instructed to produce a movement with the object that seems arbitrary or unassociated with a functional purpose. In this study, during the impoverished affordances condition, the same chopping gadget was disguised with cardboard and participants were instructed to simply push the handle down. Participants were videotaped as they reached toward the chopper in both the enriched and impoverished affordance conditions, and motion analysis technology computed variables that represented movement efficiency. The researchers found that enriched affordances had a positive effect on movement kinematics in both the poststroke and neurologically intact groups. Of greatest interest, though, was that they found that the variables reflecting smoothness of movement were significantly affected only for the poststroke group. In other words, the impact of impoverished affordances on individuals with hemiparesis is greater than the impact of impoverished affordances on individuals with intact neuromuscular function. The implication is that movement sequences that are devoid of object affordances, such as pure exercise or loose simulations of activity, are less effective than activity-based motor challenges in eliciting efficient, smooth, and coordinated movement with the paretic arm in stroke survivors.

A subsequent Level I randomized controlled trial by Trombly and Wu (1999) investigated the effect of presence or absence of an object (goal-directed action versus rote exercise). Using a counterbalanced repeated measures design, participants reached with their paretic arm to the same location under two conditions: object present, in which they reached for a self-chosen snack, and object absent, in which they reached forward with no object goal. Participants were videotaped as they reached, and motion analysis technology computed variables that represented movement efficiency. In the object-present condition, the movements were significantly faster, more forceful, smoother, and more preplanned than they were in the object-absent condition.

Trombly and Wu's findings (1999) were replicated by Wu, Trombly, Lin, and Tickle-Degnen (2000) in another study involving 14 stroke survivors with hemiparesis and 25 healthy adults. In this study, participants also were videotaped as they reached to the same location under two conditions: object present and object absent. This time, the object-present condition required participants to scoop coins off a table into their other hand, while the object-absent condition required them to reach to the same location with no object goal. The results of motion analysis computations revealed better reaching performance during the object-present condition.

In a Level I randomized controlled trial using a counterbalanced repeated-measures design, Fasoli, Trombly, Tickle-Degnen, and Verfaellie (2002) investigated the effect of verbal instructions on functional reach in stroke patients and persons without disability. For both groups, when instructions focused on task-related parameters (e.g., the location, size, or weight of the object to be lifted), arm movements were faster and more forceful than when instructions focused on internal-movement factors (e.g., the actual movements of elbow, wrist, or fingers). The clinical implication from these findings is that instead of following the practice of instructing stroke survivors to improve their movement by focusing on the intrinsic process of movement production, therapy may be more effective when it uses object affordances to guide the motor plan toward desired variables. An example is illustrated in the situation where the therapeutic goal is to encourage lateral, rather than medial, rotation of the glenohumeral joint during forward reach. Instead of directing a stroke survivor to focus on "rotating your arm out" while reaching forward in an exercise routine, the therapist would instruct the person to "pick up the phone by grasping it from its outer surface" (rather than its inner or upper surfaces, which would elicit medial rotation).

The studies just described, in which object affordances were shown to enhance the effectiveness of practice opportunities to use the paretic arm in stroke survivors, are consistent with the findings of an earlier Level II nonrandomized controlled trial (Smedley et al., 1986). This study, conducted in an inpatient rehabilitation facility in Las Vegas (notable for its population's familiarity with legalized gambling), assigned 50 stroke survivors to either standard therapy exercises or to a program in which they interacted with slot machines for the purpose of performing repeated motions with their paretic arms. The experimental group showed significantly greater improvements in outcome variables associated with range of motion, muscle strength, fine motor coordination, and gross motor coordination.

A Level I randomized controlled trial (Winstein et al., 2004) compared two experimental treatments of functional task practice (FT) and strength training (ST) to the control treatment of standard care (SC) in 64 rehabilitation inpatients with recent, first-time stroke. These researchers used the Orpington Prognostic Scale to divide participants into two levels of stroke severity (less severe and more severe) and randomly assigned participants to the three treatment groups, randomized within severity strata. All participants received customary rehabilitation interventions provided at the facility. In addition, those assigned to the FT and ST groups received additional therapy for 1 hour per day, 5 days per week over a 4-week period for a total of 20 additional therapy hours. The FT group participated in "systematic and repetitive practice of tasks that could be performed within the level of available voluntary motion," with an emphasis on providing functional goals with motivational and engaging challenges. The ST group participated in exercises to available muscles, provided according to each muscle's capacity to generate force in gravity-lessened positions, against gravity, or against resistance using free weights.

All participants were tested on three occasions: before treatment, immediately after the 4-week treatment (posttreatment), and 9 months later (long-term outcomes). On posttreatment assessment, no treatment differences were found for participants with more severe stroke impairment for any of the three types of interventions. In participants with less severe stroke impairment (67% of the total sample), significant gains were made by all three groups in pre- and posttreatment impairment scores. However, the FT and ST groups improved significantly more than the SC group on scores for impairment, strength, and function. There were no statistically significant differences between the FT and ST groups. At 9-month follow-up, among those with less severe stroke impairment, the FT group improved significantly more than either the ST or SC groups on strength (as measured by isometric torque) in upper-extremity muscles. There were no statistically significant differences between groups on other assessments. The authors reported that "intervention strategies that provide context-relevant, meaningful engagement in activities and promote self-management are more beneficial for skill acquisition and transfer than rote exercises or passive modalities" (p. 627). This explanation, with its references to Lin, Wu, Tickle-Degnen, and Coster (1997) and Ma, Trombly, and Robinson-Podolski (1999), directly supports the basic tenets of occupational therapy interventions.

Constraint-Induced Movement Therapy (CIMT)

Background Information

CIMT is a well-studied and effective treatment to improve functional arm and hand use in a small population of stroke survivors who exhibit specific motor criteria. Eligibility for participation in CIMT requires that a stroke survivor exhibit a minimum of 10° active wrist extension, 10° active thumb abduction or extension, and 10° extension in at least two additional digits with the ability to repeat these movements 3 times in 1 minute. In addition, CIMT participants also must exhibit high levels of standing balance and be able to stand from a sitting position without relying on assistance from the unaffected hand. Furthermore, CIMT participants require high levels of cognitive function and extremely high motivation to improve functional use of their paretic arm and hand (Kunkel et al., 1999). Standard CIMT protocol lasts 14 days and has two components that are both designed to promote intense, functionally oriented task practice with the paretic arm and hand. First, the person's less affected upper limb is physically constrained for 90% of waking hours by a restraining shoulder sling and/or a hand mitt. Second, the person participates in therapy sessions for 6 hours a day, 5 days per week. These sessions consist of functional task engagement with the affected arm and hand following principles of "shaping" to provide manageable but challenging task requirements. Typically, participants engage in sustained practice for 30 minutes at a time, interspersed with 20 to 30 minute rest periods (Taub et al., 1994).

CIMT has its roots in observations made during animal lesion research. In studying the effects of deafferentation to the forelimbs of experimental monkeys through dorsal rhizotomy, Taub (1976) observed that the monkeys behaved as if these limbs were paralyzed, even though the animals were capable of performing voluntary movements with the affected extremities. Taub (1976) reported his own observations, along with a review of similar findings that had been reported during the early 20th century. He coined the term "learned nonuse" to describe the phenomenon in which the monkeys developed a learned behavior of relying exclusively on a single forelimb when they were faced with an initial period of partial impairment in their ability to use the contralateral limb. Taub postulated that learned nonuse developed in response to the coupling of negative reinforcers when the monkeys unsuccessfully tried to use the affected forelimb and positive reinforcers when they successfully used compensatory behavior patterns to perform tasks unilaterally with the unimpaired forelimb. Even when the animals experienced neurological recovery, they continued this behavior of relying exclusively on the unimpaired forearm for functional performance. Taub (1976) provided evidence to support the theory of learned nonuse in experiments that restrained the unimpaired forelimbs of monkeys who had undergone lesion surgery. As predicted, when the restraining devices were removed, the experimental animals were able to use the deafferented limb and demonstrated smooth, functional motor performance.

The first clinical application to human stroke survivors was the program of "forced use." In this protocol, individuals who had sustained a stroke more than

1 year previously and met the motor criteria (described above) constrained their unaffected upper limb for 90% of waking hours over a specified period. The first clinical report (Ostendorf & Wolf, 1981) was of a single case design study of one stroke survivor with right hemiparesis. In this A-B-A design, repeated evaluations were collected during a 1-week baseline phase; a 1-week experimental phase, during which her left arm and hand were restrained; and a second 1-week follow-up baseline phase, in which the restraint was removed. The single subject exhibited increased performance speed in tests of functional activities, as well as a decreased occurrence in associated reactions and extraneous movements of her right arm and hand. In addition, during the follow-up baseline phase, the woman reported an increase in the repertoire of functional tasks she could perform with her right arm and hand.

In the following two decades, Taub, Uswatte, and Pidikiti (1999) added the component of supervised practice sessions, using the technique of shaping to gradually refine task demands and coined the term "constraint-induced movement therapy" to describe this combined intervention of intensive practice and constraint to the unaffected upper limb. The researchers also developed specific assessments to measure treatment outcomes. The Arm Motor Assessment Test (AMAT; Kopp et al., 1997) and the Wolf Motor Function Test (WMFT; Morris et al., 2001; Wolf et al., 2001) evaluate functional motor performance of a paretic upper limb. The Motor Activity Log (MAL; Taub et al., 1993) assesses a stroke survivor's own perceptions of how well and how often he or she uses the paretic upper limb during daily activities.

Recent Evidence

CIMT generated considerable interest in the rehabilitation community and several Level III, noncontrolled studies tested its effectiveness in small samples. In 2002, a Level V review (Wolf, Blanton, Baer, Breshears, & Butler, 2002) reported findings from 22 independent trials. The studies measured clinical outcomes with the AMAT, MAL, and WMFT. In addition,

researchers used TMS to quantify changes in neural reorganization associated with the motor improvements exhibited by stroke survivors who participated in CIMT.

The Extremity Constraint-Induced Therapy Evaluation (EXCITE) trial, a prospective, single blind, randomized, multisite clinical trial conducted at 7 U.S. academic medical centers between January 2001 and January 2003, is the largest systematic outcomes study in the history of stroke rehabilitation in the United States. Through recruitment from 247 facilities spanning the 7 participating sites, 3,626 individuals were screened to identify 222 stroke survivors who met standard CIMT criteria. These criteria, and the extensive assessments administered to all participants in the EXCITE trial, are described by Winstein and colleagues (2003). All participants were 3- to 9-months poststroke.

The 222 selected participants were randomly assigned to either a control or experimental group. Control group members continued to receive usual and customary care that ranged from no treatment to participation in various occupational therapy and physical therapy approaches at outpatient hospital settings, at home, or in day treatment programs. Participants in the intervention group were taught to apply a safety mitt to their less involved hand, with the goal of wearing the mitt for 90% of waking hours over a 2-week period, including weekends. On each weekday of the 2-week period, while continuing to wear the restraining mitt, these participants participated in 6 hours per day of shaping and standard task training using the paretic arm and hand. Standard task practice consisted of functional activities performed continuously for a period of 15 to 20 minutes. Following standard CIMT protocol, participants followed several behavioral techniques to enhance their use of the mitt during hours outside the training sessions. These included use of a behavioral contract, caregiver contract, and daily schedule report. In addition, a mitt compliance device, which consisted of a sensor and timer within the mitt, provided objective information to the researchers about the amount of time the mitt was worn within specified periods. Furthermore, homework tasks were routinely assigned by therapists for participants to actively practice between weekday shaping sessions.

Participants in both groups were tested on five occasions by trained, blinded evaluators at baseline; immediately posttreatment; and 4 months, 8 months, and 12 months posttreatment (Wolf et al., 2006). Those who received CIMT were followed again 2 years after completing the intervention (Wolf et al., 2008). Measurements included the WMFT; MAL; and the Stroke Impact Scale (SIS), a self-report assessing health-related quality of life for stroke survivors.

The findings provide support for the efficacy of CIMT for improving arm and hand motor function in stroke survivors who meet criteria to participate in this intervention. From baseline to 12 months, the CIMT group demonstrated significantly greater improvements than the control group in WMFT performance time, MAL amount of use, MAL quality of movement, and self-perceived hand function on the SIS (Level I; Wolf et al., 2006). The achievements shown by CIMT participants were maintained on testing 2 years after intervention (Level I; Wolf et al., 2008). Significant improvements were noted at 2-year follow-up on WMFT strength tasks and in several subtests on the SIS. These results are consistent with findings of a previous study of task-related training (Level I; Winstein et al. 2004) that, among stroke survivors who learn to actively use their paretic arm during functional daily activities, there is potential to continually improve arm and hand strength for years after completing a therapeutic intervention.

Adaptations to CIMT

CIMT has attracted considerable attention from rehabilitation professionals. Because the intensity of the program is a source of pragmatic concern, several adaptations to CIMT have been proposed and evaluated. The goal is to find a level of modification that will decrease costs and improve accessibility to more stroke survivors while maintaining highly beneficial outcomes. A Level I randomized controlled trial comparing two small groups of CIMT participants receiving either 6 hours per day or 3 hours per day of shaping therapy

(Sterr et al., 2002) in a standard CIMT protocol found statistically significant improvements on the MAL and WMFT for both groups; however, the improvements shown by the 6-hour-per-day group were significantly greater than those shown by the group receiving fewer hours of supervised motor practice. Flinn, Schamburg, Fetrow, and Flanigan (2005) modified standard CIMT protocol by shortening the program duration from 14 to 8 days and by providing 3.5 hours of treatment per day. In their Level III study, they collected data using the MAL, the WFMT, and the Canadian Occupational Performance Measure (COPM). The 11 participants in this study exhibited statistically significant improvement in MAL scores on testing 7 days after treatment ended and at a 4- to 6-month follow-up, as well as significant improvements in COPM Satistifaction Scores at the 4- to 6-month follow-up. Flinn and colleagues elucidated two important practical considerations that may potentially limit widespread use of standard CIMT protocols with large numbers of stroke survivors who meet CIMT criteria. First, even after following recommended behavioral incentives to maximize compliance with the recommended mitt-wearing schedule of 90% of waking hours, these researchers found that actual mitt wearing ranged from 1.2% to 79%, with an average of 48.9% of waking hours. It is possible that to fully comply with a standard CIMT mitt-wearing schedule, it is necessary for participants to have the added safety (and psychological security) of a full-time companion. Second, they found that fatigue was an issue for several participants and that only 4 of the 11 participants in their modified program were able to tolerate even the abbreviated 3.5 hours of intensive task practice per day.

Flinn and colleagues suggested that group interactions during CIMT shaping sessions may be beneficial to the rehabilitation process. Brogardh and Sjölund (2006) explored this further in a Level III study assessing a group program in which 2 to 3 patients worked with a single therapist for 6 hours per day of treatment for 12 days, in addition to following the standard CIMT protocol for wearing a hand mitt for 90% of waking hours. Their findings of statistically significant improvements in motor performance on two measures of arm and hand function provide support for the efficacy of providing shaping training in a group setting.

Page and colleagues (Levine & Page, 2004) proposed an alternative to CIMT that conforms to the practical realities of current reimbursement regulations for stroke rehabilitation in the United States. In their protocol, which they named modified CIMT (mCIMT), stroke survivors who meet CIMT criteria wear a restrictive mitt for only 5 hours per day, 5 days per week for a 10-week duration, and participate in practice sessions that are comparable to traditional outpatient rehabilitation therapy sessions (usually 30-minute sessions 3 days per week). An important practical benefit to mCIMT is that participants are more likely to comply with the mitt-wearing schedule while still being able to continue their engagement in work, volunteer, or leisure activities. In a series of studies enrolling both stroke survivors and adults with hemiparesis following traumatic brain injury, Page and colleagues provided Level I support for mCIMT's effectiveness (Page, Levine, Leonard, Szaflarski, & Kissela, 2008; Page, Sisto, Levine, & McGrath, 2004) and demonstrated *f*MRI evidence for cortical reorganization accompanying motor improvements in patients who have completed the mCIMT protocol (Szaflarski et al., 2006). Independent investigators have supported these findings in a Level I study of elderly stroke survivors who participated in a 3-week program of mCIMT (Wu, Chen, Tsai, Lin, & Chou, 2007). They demonstrated significant improvements in kinematic variables of reach and grasp using motion analysis technology to compare performance by 3-week mCIMT participants with a control group of stroke survivors who received traditional rehabilitation intervention.

In summary, the collective body of research about CIMT and its various adaptations provides direct support for the essential occupational therapy tenet that opportunities for practice within the natural context of activity engagement are critical and necessary for improving motor skill. Interventions that increase a client's active involvement and creative problem solving will enhance the amount and quality of practice

and ultimately result in more significant improvements in motor performance.

Robot-Assisted Therapy

Recent advances in robotic technology have created new possibilities for providing stroke survivors with opportunities for high-intensity, active, task-oriented, repetitive upper-limb movement practice, as well as objective, reliable monitoring of patient progress (Prange, Jannink, Groothuis-Oudshoorn, Hermens, & Ijzerman, 2006). In robot-aided therapy, a patient's paretic upper limb is placed on a handle that he or she moves to reach a series of target locations that are illustrated on a computer screen. Depending on each person's performance, the robot provides either partial assistance or graded resistance to the stroke survivor's own active movements. On the basis of continuous, objective monitoring, the robot also controls and quantifies the intensity of practice (Fasoli, Krebs, Stein, Frontera, & Hogan, 2003). Although engineers have designed robotic technology to train movement at every possible segment of the upper limb, clinical studies published to date have assessed only the efficacy of robotic devices that train shoulder and elbow movements. A Level I systematic review (Prange et al., 2006) of robot-aided therapy for upper-limb recovery after stroke found eight studies that met its methodological criteria. Six of these studies had a pre- and posttreatment measurement design for robot-aided therapy. Although several of them used random assignment of participants to two different types of robotic interventions, they did not compare participants to a control group of stroke survivors who received a non robotic treatment or no treatment at all. Collectively, these studies reported both short-term and long-term effects of robot-aided therapy that were clinically significant. Two of the studies were experimental trials with pre- and posttreatment measurements of both an experimental and a control group, and one of these was a Level I randomized controlled trial. The randomized controlled trial (Lum, Burgar, Shor, Majmundar, & Van der Loos, 2002) included in the systematic review randomly allocated 27 participants with chronic hemiparesis (more than 6 months poststroke) to the experimental robot group or to a control group in which the stroke survivors received NDT targeting proximal upper limb function and 5 minutes of exposure to the robot in each session (to offset a possible placebo effect). All participants received 24 1-hour sessions over 2 months. Clinical evaluations, conducted by a therapist blinded to group assignments, were conducted midway through treatment, after treatment, and at a 6-month follow-up. Compared with the control group, the robot-aided therapy group had larger gains in Fugl-Meyer scores at 1-month and 2-month testing, but not at the 6-month follow-up. The experimental group also showed significantly greater improvements in strength and in extent of forward reach after 2 months and in Functional Independence Measure (FIM) scores at the 6-month follow-up.

In summary, for stroke survivors who are unable to independently perform meaningful, repetitive activities with their paretic arm and hand, robot-aided training provides benefits of intensity and repeatability of practice that cannot be replicated by a therapist giving hand-over-hand assistance during functional task performance. Currently, the technology is commercially available, but cost limits its use in most rehabilitation facilities.

A review of the collective literature about robotics, CIMT, and other research related to improving motor function after stroke yields findings from occupational therapy researchers and other professionals that support the use of activity-based interventions with familiar objects in therapeutic interventions to improve motor skills in stroke survivors.

Intervention to Improve Cognitive, Perceptual, and Praxis Skills

Cognitive and perceptual impairments significantly affect activities of daily living (ADLs) and instrumental activities of daily living function (Lincoln, Drummond, & Berman, 1997; Zinn et al., 2004). Four Level I systematic reviews (Bowen, Lincoln, & Dewey, 2002; Ma & Trombly, 2002; Majid, Lincoln, & Weyman, 2000; Steultjens et al., 2003) agreed that evidence to support the efficacy of occupational therapy or other interventions in improving cognitive and per-

ceptual skills in stroke survivors is limited. This includes the areas of memory, attention, and executive function. There is evidence, however, for the effectiveness of occupational therapy with regard to cognitive and perceptual skills in stroke survivors in the areas of apraxia and spatial neglect.

Apraxia, associated with left hemisphere pathology, refers to difficulties in executing learned movement sequences beyond limitations that could be explained by weakness, lack of coordination, sensory loss, comprehension deficits, memory, or motivation. The available evidence supports training in the use of compensatory strategies for clients with apraxia to achieve improvements in ADL function. Specifically, the occupational therapist determines how the client's deficit is impeding one of three stages required in motor planning of selected functional tasks: initiation, execution, or ongoing control. Following this, the occupational therapist teaches the client a compensatory strategy, such as verbalizing the sequence during activity performance or viewing pictures that illustrate the steps required for task execution. The therapeutic goal is to improve functioning in spite of the presence of impairment in motor planning (van Heugten et al., 1998). Evidence from both a single group pre–post design (van Heugten et al., 1998) and a randomized controlled trial (Donkervoort, Dekker, Stehmann-Saris, Deelman, 2001) indicates that this intervention results in statistically significant improvements in ADL function as measured by the Barthel Index. A subsequent Level III (pretest–posttest) study with 29 patients provided support for the long-term and generalized effects of this compensatory strategy intervention. For stroke survivors with apraxia who were tested in their own homes after 8 weeks of training and again 7 weeks after training ended, the statistically significant improvements in ADL function made during training were maintained on retesting. In addition, patients were able to generalize their learned strategies to other tasks at home that they had never practiced during the intervention (Geusgens, van Heugten, Cooijmans, Jolles, & van den Heuvel, 2006). Although apraxia is associated with other cognitive impairments, such as language comprehension, cognitive orientation, and short-term memory, this intervention to develop compensatory strategies is not influenced by cognitive comorbidities (van Heugten, Dekker, Deelman, Stehmann-Saris, & Kinebanian, 2000).

Results of two studies provide additional support for the efficacy of task-based training to improve specific skills in stroke patients with motor apraxia. In a Level II nonrandomized controlled trial, Goldenberg, Hentze, and Hermsdörfer (2004) investigated whether patients with motor apraxia would perform better when using real tools than when pantomiming the use of tools. The participating stroke patients demonstrated the use of 12 tools under three conditions: pantomime with visual input (a photograph of a tool), pantomime with visual and tactile input (a photograph of a tool and a wooden implement resembling the handle of the tool), and real use. All patients performed significantly better under real use than under either of the other conditions.

In another Level II nonrandomized controlled trial, Poole (1998) studied the effect of motor apraxia on the ability of stroke patients to learn and retain a functional sequencing task, one-handed shoe tying. The stroke patients without apraxia performed significantly better than the stroke patients with apraxia on both learning and retention. However, 4 of the 5 participants with apraxia were able to retain the task after a 5-minute delay.

Spatial neglect is a disorder in attending to stimuli presented in the space contralateral to a brain lesion, beyond motor and sensory deficits (Heilman & Valenstein, 1979). A variety of names for it are used interchangeably, including *unilateral neglect, hemi-neglect, hemi-inattention, scanning deficit,* and *spatial awareness disorders.* A growing body of evidence supports the use of interventions designed to enhance patients' awareness of this deficit with follow-up training in compensatory strategies (Fischer, Gauggel, & Trexler, 2004).

A Level I systematic review of cognitive rehabilitation for spatial neglect following stroke (Bowen et al., 2002) limited inclusion to controlled trials in which at least 75% of the sample were stroke patients. Fifteen studies by neuropsychologists and by occupational therapists met these criteria. The pooled evidence supports the efficacy of cognitive rehabilitation in improving performance on paper-and-pencil cancellation tests, but it does not provide strong support for generalization to performance of daily activities. The reviewers acknowledge that the shortage of support may be due to methodological factors. In particular, currently available measures of disability may not be sensitive enough to detect change as a result of improvements in spatial awareness. Further randomized controlled trials are needed, using functional outcome measures designed to assess changes in activity performance that are affected by improved spatial awareness. Some preliminary findings indicate that the Assessment of Motor and Process Skills (AMPS), a tool designed from an occupational therapy perspective, may be more appropriate than traditional neuropsychological tests as an outcome measure of functional improvements resulting from therapeutic interventions (Linden, Boschian, Eker, Schalen, & Nordstrom, 2005).

Transfer of Training

Rehabilitation professionals from several disciplines agree that "transfer," or "transfer of training," is a critical goal when providing strategy-based interventions to stroke survivors with impairments in process skills. Transfer of training, or generalization, is a person's successful application of a learned strategy to new tasks that he or she has not directly practiced. A Level I systematic review of transfer in cognitive rehabilitation (Geusgens, Winkens, van Heugten, Jolles, & van den Heuvel, 2007) found 41 separate studies that met inclusion criteria of measuring transfer outcomes of cognitive strategy training in adults surviving stroke or other brain injury. Interventions focused primarily on the cognitive domains of neglect, memory, and language, but strategy training was also used to improve information processing, problem solving or executive functioning, and attention. Of the eight studies that specified the professional affiliation of the trainers, 75% used occupational therapists to provide the cognitive strategy intervention. This is not surprising because occupational therapy's focus on improving functional task performance is consistent with an emphasis on generalization of learned skills rather than on outcomes measured by impairment-based evaluations. This systematic review's finding that most studies reported positive results with regard to transfer of training effects supports the use of cognitive strategy interventions within the naturalistic context of activity performance to improve functional performance by stroke survivors with impairments in process skills. This finding, in contrast to Bowen and colleagues (2002), supports the use of everyday activities rather than paper-and-pencil tasks as a way of developing generalizable cognitive strategies in stroke survivors.

Improvement in Activity and Role Performance

Participation in activities and role performance are key outcomes in stroke rehabilitation. Occupational therapy practitioners play a critical role in restoring independence, even in patients who are unable to achieve improvements in motor status. In this realm too, a moderate-sized body of evidence supports the efficacy of occupational therapy intervention. Three Level I systematic reviews specific to occupational therapy analyzed the evidence (Legg et al., 2006; Steultjens et al., 2003; Trombly & Ma, 2002), as did five multidisciplinary practice guidelines (Gresham et al., 1995; New Zealand Guidelines Group, 2003; Ottawa Panel, 2006; Scottish Intercollegiate Guidelines Network, 2002; SCORE, 2007).

It is well recognized that as members of the interdisciplinary stroke rehabilitation team, occupational therapy practitioners help enhance patients' functional independence, and their contributions are well recognized. In a retrospective Level III study with a before-and-after design, Roth et al., (1998) compared improvements in activity performance by two groups of stroke patients who had undergone inpatient rehabilitation: those who experienced reduction in stroke-related impairments and those whose impairments remained unchanged. Although 85% of the patients in this study made no substantial impairment-related gains, both groups experienced significant improvement in functional performance as measured by the FIM; at discharge, differences between the two groups in scores on that measure were relatively small. These findings support the value of occupational therapy interventions to improve task-performance skills, in spite of residual stroke-related impairments.

Bode, Heinemann, Semik, and Mallinson (2004) conducted a Level II cohort study at 13 facilities to examine factors of inpatient rehabilitation programs that influenced functional outcomes in stroke survivors beyond what would have been predicted by scores on the FIM on admission. They found two significant factors that influenced gains in self-care: longer lengths of stay and more intensive function-focused occupational therapy.

In another Level II cohort study of inpatient rehabilitation, Lenze and colleagues (2004) compared functional outcomes on the basis of patients' attendance levels in physical and occupational therapy programs. Patients with good participation in therapy programs demonstrated significantly higher changes in motor scores on the FIM than patients with poor participation. This finding lends further support to the efficacy of occupational therapy services in improving activity performance after stroke.

A solid body of international research evidence supports the efficacy of occupational therapy intervention during the phase of continuing adjustment. Outpatient Service Trialists (2004), in a Level I systematic review of randomized trials assessing outcomes of rehabilitation services for stroke rehabilitation patients living at home, reported consistent support for the efficacy of occupational therapy in improving functional performance in both basic and extended ADLs. This review, using the strategy approved by the Cochrane Controlled Trials Register (Higgins & Green, 2005), included four studies of multidisciplinary team programs, two studies of home-based physical therapy services, and six studies of occupational therapy interventions.

In a Level I systematic review and meta-analysis included in the Cochrane Collaboration database, Legg et al. (2006), identified 64 randomized controlled trials that were potentially eligible for review, but finally reviewed 10 studies with 1,348 participants. The identified studies were targeted at improving ADLs. The results indicated that stroke patients who had received treatment from an occupational therapist were more independent in ADLs (feeding, dressing, bathing, toileting, moving about) and more likely to maintain these abilities than stroke patients who had not received treatment from an occupational therapist.

In a Level I meta-analysis of 8 randomized controlled trials of community-based occupational therapy for stroke patients that encompassed 1,143 patients, Walker and colleagues (2004) found that occupational therapy was associated with statistically significant improvements in ADLs and participation in leisure pursuits. These studies were conducted in Great Britain, where delivery systems for outpatient and home-based occupational therapy services provide greater ease of randomly assigning stroke survivors to occupational therapy treatment and control groups. Also, community-based occupational therapy services are financially supported by the national health care system.

The occupational therapy services reported in the eight studies covered by Walker and colleagues (2004) mirror the interventions described in this Guideline. Using individualized, top-down assessment, the occupational therapists identify a combination of client skills, activity demands, and environmental factors that impede task performance and are amenable to change. The therapists then systematically develop practice opportunities, activity adaptations, and environmental modifications that enable each stroke survivor to meet self-selected goals. Level I studies reviewed by Walker and colleagues support the efficacy of this approach in improving the specific ability to get dressed (Walker, Drummond, & Lincoln, 1996), decreasing caregiver strain (Walker, Gladman, Lincoln, Siemonsma, & Whiteley, 1999), enhancing scores on the Barthel Index of self-care independence (Walker et al., 1999), and improving scores on assessments of extended ADL (Logan, Ahern, Gladman, & Lincoln, 1997).

Some research supports the efficacy of occupational therapy intervention in improving leisure participation (e.g., Drummond and Walker [1995], a Level I study included in Walker and colleagues [2004]). However, Parker and colleagues (2001), in another Level I study in the review by Walker and colleagues (2004), found

no indication that occupational therapy with a specific focus on leisure activities was more effective than a conventional, holistic occupational therapy program in enhancing the participation of stroke survivors in leisure pursuits. A Level I randomized controlled trial conducted after the review by Walker and colleagues provided support for the efficacy of targeted occupational therapy intervention to increase outdoor mobility in people after stroke. Logan and colleagues (2004) used individualized occupational therapy with stroke survivors in the postrehabilitation stage to enhance *outdoor mobility*, defined as the ability to use local public transportation or resume driving. Occupational therapy services yielded significant differences between experimental and control group members in community participation, as measured by the number of excursions outside the home per month.

Research indicates, however, that activity and participation outcomes of community-based occupational therapy intervention may not be maintained indefinitely. Two Level I follow-up studies included in the review by Walker and colleagues (2004; Gilbertson, Langhorne, Walker, Allen, & Murray, 2000; Logan et al., 1997) showed that significant differences between participants in experimental and control groups that were present 3 months after intervention were no longer apparent after 6 months.

These findings support the need for targeted, follow-up occupational therapy to maintain independence and role engagement among community-dwelling stroke survivors.

Summary of the Evidence

The evidence-based literature review yielded many high-quality human studies (Appendix B). Of the 97 studies included in the review, nearly two-thirds (62) of the articles reviewed were at the highest level of evidence (Level I), and 17 of the articles were at the second highest level of evidence (Level II). Twenty-two of the Level I studies included in the review were systematic reviews and meta-analyses covering a variety of topics related to occupational therapy and stroke.

Several limitations of the individual studies included in the review need to be kept in mind. These limitations include small sample sizes, possible attention or selection bias, co-intervention, possible spontaneous recovery, lack of randomization and control groups, ceiling effect on learning task, large number of outcomes, and a period of treatment that may be too short to evaluate intervention effectiveness. Limitations specific to the systematic reviews include the possibility that trials included in a review may not be comparable with variations in interventions across countries.

The review also included eight additional animal studies. Four studies were Level I and four were Level II studies. Limitations of the animal studies include small sample sizes, the possibility that lesions were not large enough to allow for the differentiation of effects of various measures, and the possibility that motor skill measures were not sensitive enough to detect subtle differences in behavior.

In summary, the available research evidence supports occupational therapy's use of individualized, activity-based interventions to promote neural plasticity, enhance motor control in patients who exhibit neural sparing of some efferent pathways, and enhance occupational function, regardless of motor recovery. More research is needed to support the impact of specific occupational therapy interventions on improving cognitive and perceptual skills. In particular, these studies need to examine measurable, function-based outcomes, such as caregiver burden, activity independence, and caregiver- or survivor-based reports about participation and quality of life.

The research support is strong for occupational therapy's impact on occupational performance and participation. However, longitudinal studies are needed to assess long-term outcomes in stroke survivors. Failure to find that occupational therapy–related outcomes are sustained indefinitely should not necessarily be interpreted as a limitation of the interventions. Rather, just as routine follow-up visits to physicians are considered to be essential, intermittent occupational therapy "check-ups" may prove to be a valid, cost-effective component to ongoing, adequate health care for the stroke population.

Implications of the Evidence-Based Literature Review for Occupational Therapy Research, Education, and Practice

Implications for Research

The occupational therapy profession has a primary need for a cadre of researchers whose focus is developing, securing funding for, and implementing clinical outcome studies of occupational therapy interventions with stroke survivors. The challenges of conducting controlled group studies with stroke survivors are significant, as it is difficult to recruit participants when similar services are available through standard clinical programs. In addition, the individualized nature of occupational therapy interventions makes it difficult to assess the efficacy of a standard research protocol. To overcome the ethical constraints of denying treatment to control group participants, we need to expand the number of Level I studies that recruit stroke survivors who have previously completed their initial poststroke rehabilitation, and provide interventions in community-based, outpatient settings. Instead of comparing isolated treatments to one another, to preserve the holistic nature of occupational therapy interventions, control group participants receiving no occupational therapy should be compared to experimental group participants to whom expert clinicians are providing client-centered programs based on individualized, standard assessments. The outcomes of interest in these studies would be scores on assessments of functional performance, as well as participation in daily life and community activities.

In addition, academic researchers must work in partnership with clinicians and administrators to implement Level II outcome studies of inpatient, outpatient, and home-based rehabilitation. Specifically, researchers need to assess the effectiveness of interventions designed to improve motor, cognitive, and perceptual function, as measured by clients' own reflections about their performance of daily activities. Many occupational therapists have experimented with taping and various types of spasticity-reducing splints for patients with hypertonicity to improve comfort and functional use of the paretic arm. Researchers within our profession need to investigate the efficacy of these interventions using well-selected outcome variables.

The growing body of evidence in support of CIMT, largely by researchers external to the occupational therapy profession, provides support for occupational therapy's foundational focus on the value of activity-based intervention. Most experts agree that it is not the constraint itself but rather the enhanced opportunities for practice using the paretic upper limb that contribute to improvements in functional performance after CIMT. Occupational therapy researchers need to take the next step and assess whether equivalent doses of engagement in bilateral motor activities yield similar positive outcomes as constraint-induced unilateral motor activity with the paretic arm and hand. In addition, we need to follow up on the outcome studies done to date that assess the efficacy of occupational therapy interventions in enhancing occupational performance in stroke survivors with cognitive and perceptual impairments.

Occupational therapy researchers can benefit by developing partnerships with investigators in other disciplines. Collaborative investigations with neuroscientists will be critical for assessing evidence of neural reorganization in patients who have developed enhanced motor or process skills after specific occupational therapy interventions. Robotics and functional electrical stimulation are two areas of intervention with a growing body of support that is generated primarily by researchers in disciplines outside occupational therapy. Occupational therapists should collaborate with these researchers to develop studies that assess the efficacy of combining individualized, task-based interventions with the two modalities. Also, occupational therapists can work with computer engineers toward determining ways to individualize video game and virtual-reality technology to provide individualized therapeutic challenges to motor and process skills.

Finally, we need to explore the efficacy of expanding the scope of occupational therapy interventions with stroke survivors beyond hospital settings to ongoing community-based interventions. On the basis of models of care reported from Great Britain, occupational therapy researchers can undertake a longitudinal study of stroke survivors in which participants in the treatment group have semiannual short-term interventions by occupational therapists. Such a study would be critical in determining if this alternative model of care is effective in maintaining independence, expanding activity engagement, and enhancing health-related quality of life in stroke survivors over the course of their lives. Positive results would be important to lobbying efforts that inform national health policy and third-party reimbursement of occupational therapy services.

Implications for Education

A basic understanding of contemporary neuroscience is critical to interpreting and applying studies of brain plasticity. Occupational therapy curricula must continue to include course work which ensures that graduates are competent consumers of the neuroscience literature.

Several neurofacilitative approaches to treatment for patients recovering from stroke and brain injury were introduced in the mid-20th century, one after another, but countless attempts to establish evidence of their efficacy have been unsuccessful. Current textbooks and curricula continue to present a variety of approaches, implying that each practitioner should choose the approach that appeals to his or her interest. Educators should seriously evaluate the profession's framework for teaching students the knowledge and skills they will need to provide evidence-based interventions to stroke survivors. Educators must assume the ongoing responsibility of monitoring the methods and findings of published research studies and design their course content accordingly. The profession's national accreditation standards for academic programs include the requirement that graduates be skilled in administering and interpreting findings from standardized assessments. Educators are responsible for continually monitoring which evaluation tools are most commonly used in published research studies for the purpose of updating which evaluation procedures will be included in lectures and labs related to stroke intervention.

Finally, occupational therapy graduates must have skills to provide ongoing community-based programs to stroke survivors in both individual and group settings. The emphasis should be on helping people maintain healthy habits and patterns for preventing secondary impairments and for staying actively involved in multiple life roles.

Implications for Practice

The growing evidence supporting the human brain's capacity to reorganize itself after injury is of critical importance to occupational therapy intervention with stroke survivors. Occupational therapists must routinely and carefully assess patients for signs of specific motor capacity on the affected side and develop individualized, activity-based practice challenges that capitalize on any available movement.

At the same time, occupational therapists must understand that regardless of the extent of primary motor return, secondary impairments, such as postural misalignment and loss of muscle length, will interfere with a patient's ultimate capacity to functionally use a paretic arm or leg. Most of these impairments are directly related to immobility and awkward postures. Therefore, in addition to fostering mobility as soon as medically feasible after the stroke, occupational therapy practitioners must teach patients and their families daily techniques for stretching spastic muscles and maintaining healthy postural alignment when lying in bed, sitting, and standing.

Occupational therapists must understand the importance of using standardized assessments to evaluate the outcomes of their interventions. A typical stroke survivor receives interventions at multiple sites from multiple therapists. Consistent use of standardized assessments enhances continuity of care and allows for retrospective analysis of individual and aggregate patient outcomes. In addition, occupational therapists must assess the functional impact of their interventions using standardized assessments and focused interview questions to determine changes in occupational performance, physical comfort, use of the paretic arm and leg, and role participation.

Animal and human studies provide a body of evidence that learned nonuse is a significant factor limiting function in a percentage of stroke survivors who fail to use their available motor capacity. Occupational therapists need to be aware that overemphasis on early training in one-handed techniques for self-care activities can contribute to learned nonuse.

Still, solid research supports occupational therapy interventions targeted at improving patients' abilities to perform ADLs. Such interventions have positive and significant outcomes related to general health, patients' mood, and caregivers' health satisfaction. Therefore, occupational therapists must use their professional expertise to tailor self-care strategies that capitalize on each patient's individual motor capacities. There cannot be a standard method for teaching stroke survivors to dress or feed themselves. Rather, occupational therapists must apply their knowledge of human movement to create adaptations that challenge each person's motor capacities while allowing for their independent performance.

A significant body of evidence supports the value of activity-based practice rather than repetitive movement in improving motor skills in stroke survivors. Occupational therapists must use skill and creativity in designing activities that motivate patients to practice with full effort and attention. In popular culture, video games and virtual-reality activities have captured widespread interest from consumers. It behooves occupational therapists to incorporate these modalities into individualized activity challenges for stroke patients.

The evidence for interventions to improve cognitive and perceptual skills in stroke survivors also supports the use of activity-based practice. In this realm, the key distinction between occupational therapy practitioners and other professionals is the practitioners' emphasis on occupational performance as a treatment outcome. When providing these interventions, occupational therapy practitioners must continue to focus on how their interventions will directly affect self-care, instrumental activities of daily living, leisure, social participation, and work-related performance.

Occupational therapy practitioners must acknowledge that to attain sufficient amounts of task-related practice, stroke survivors must apply newly emerging skills in multiple contexts, above and beyond clinical therapy sessions. Accordingly, occupational therapy intervention must entail structured follow-up assignments in which clients actively apply their motor, cognitive, and social coping skills. Furthermore, clients must feel accountable for practicing on their own and for taking responsibility to develop creative ways to expand their repertoire of activity performance. Standard educational practices, such as behavioral contracts, therapy notebooks, homework assignments, and ongoing logs or homework check sheets can be routine components of occupational therapy intervention at all stages of stroke rehabilitation.

Finally, with expanding life expectancies after stroke, many stroke survivors would benefit from access to short-term occupational therapy services throughout their lives. Although such services are not specifically documented through research to date, occupational therapists need to find mechanisms for cost-effectively offering their services in community settings. In the long run, regularly scheduled occupational therapy check-ups could save health care dollars by minimizing secondary impairments and keeping people active and independent, thus enhancing health-related quality of life.

In summary, the research evidence supports the importance of individualized intervention. No two stroke survivors are the same. The occupational therapist must consider myriad factors with each client and tailor the interventions according to the person's remaining skills, potential for improvement, personal motivations, and contextual influences. The goal of occupational therapy for stroke survivors must be to help each person reach his or her unique potential for moving, thinking, performing daily activities, and participating in an active, healthy lifestyle.

■ ■ ■

Appendix A.
Preparation and Qualifications of Occupational Therapists and Occupational Therapy Assistants

Who Are Occupational Therapists?

To practice as an occupational therapist, the individual trained in the United States

- Has graduated from an occupational therapy program accredited by the Accreditation Council for Occupational Therapy Education (ACOTE®) or predecessor organizations;
- Has successfully completed a period of supervised fieldwork experience required by the recognized educational institution where the applicant met the academic requirements of an educational program for occupational therapists that is accredited by ACOTE or predecessor organizations;
- Has passed a nationally recognized entry-level examination for occupational therapists; and
- Fulfills state requirements for licensure, certification, or registration.

Educational Programs for the Occupational Therapist

These include the following:

- Biological, physical, social, and behavioral sciences
- Basic tenets of occupational therapy
- Occupational therapy theoretical perspectives
- Screening and evaluation
- Formulation and implementation of an intervention plan
- Context of service delivery
- Management of occupational therapy services (master's level)
- Leadership and management (doctoral level)

- Use of research
- Professional ethics, values, and responsibilities.

The fieldwork component of the program is designed to develop competent, entry-level, generalist occupational therapists by providing experience with a variety of clients across the life span and in a variety of settings. Fieldwork is integral to the program's curriculum design and includes an in-depth experience in delivering occupational therapy services to clients, focusing on the application of purposeful and meaningful occupation and/or research, administration, and management of occupational therapy services. The fieldwork experience is designed to promote clinical reasoning and reflective practice, to transmit the values and beliefs that enable ethical practice, and to develop professionalism and competence in career responsibilities. Doctoral-level students must also complete a doctoral experiential component designed to develop advanced skills beyond a generalist level.

Who Are Occupational Therapy Assistants?

To practice as an occupational therapy assistant, the individual trained in the United States

- Has graduated from an occupational therapy assistant program accredited by ACOTE or predecessor organizations;
- Has successfully completed a period of supervised fieldwork experience required by the recognized educational institution where the

applicant met the academic requirements of an educational program for occupational therapy assistants that is accredited by ACOTE or predecessor organizations;

- Has passed a nationally recognized entry-level examination for occupational therapy assistants; and
- Fulfills state requirements for licensure, certification, or registration.

Educational Programs for the Occupational Therapy Assistant

These include the following:
- Biological, physical, social, and behavioral sciences
- Basic tenets of occupational therapy
- Screening and assessment
- Intervention and implementation
- Context of service delivery
- Assistance in management of occupational therapy services
- Professional literature
- Professional ethics, values, and responsibilities.

The fieldwork component of the program is designed to develop competent, entry-level, generalist occupa-tional therapy assistants by providing experience with a variety of clients across the life span and in a variety of settings. Fieldwork is integral to the program's curriculum design and includes an in-depth experience in delivering occupational therapy services to clients, focusing on the application of purposeful and meaningful occupation. The fieldwork experience is designed to promote clinical reasoning appropriate to the occupational therapy assistant role, to transmit the values and beliefs that enable ethical practice, and to develop professionalism and competence in career responsibilities.

Regulation of Occupational Therapy Practice

All occupational therapists and occupational therapy assistants must practice under federal and state law. Currently, 50 states, the District of Columbia, Puerto Rico, and Guam have enacted laws regulating the practice of occupational therapy.

Note. The majority of this information is taken from the *Accreditation Standards for a Doctoral-Degree-Level Educational Program for the Occupational Therapist* (AOTA, 2007a), *Accreditation Standards for a Master's-Degree-Level Educational Program for the Occupational Therapist* (AOTA, 2007b), and *Accreditation Standards for an Educational Program for the Occupational Therapy Assistant* (AOTA, 2007c).

Appendix B.
Evidence Tables

Evidence Table on Central Nervous System Plasticity: Animal Studies

Author/Year	Study Objectives	Level/Design/Participants	Intervention & Outcome Measures	Results	Limitations
Biernaskie & Corbett (2001)	Assess effects of environmental enrichment on dendritic reorganization in intact hemisphere and on functional recovery	II—Nonrandomized controlled trial $N = 57$ Sprague-Dawley rats; assigned to intervention or control groups	Researchers induced focal ischemia in or performed sham surgery on rats. Fifteen days later, they assigned rats to ischemia plus enrichment, ischemia plus standard housing, sham plus enrichment, or sham plus standard housing. Enrichment involved giving rats rehabilitative training 5 days per week for 9 weeks and housing them in groups in large cages equipped with various objects for exploration (e.g., plastic tubing, rope). Cages were cleaned 2 times per week and objects were rearranged at those times. Outcomes: • Reaching ability (staircase skilled–reaching test) • Use of wall contact with ipsilateral forelimb for postural support (videotape) • Beam-walking ability (foot faults and latency to cross beam) • Dendritic arborization (Golgi-Cox procedure)	Ischemic-enriched rats performed significantly better than ischemic-nonenriched rats in reaching ability. Ischemic rats showed significantly greater reliance on wall contact with ipsilateral forelimb for postural support than sham rats. Ischemic-enriched rats became indistinguishable from sham rats in beam walking. Ischemic-enriched rats had significantly greater dendritic arbors in undamaged contralateral motor cortex than other groups of rats.	Lack of randomization

Reference: Biernaskie, J., & Corbett, D. (2001). Enriched rehabilitative training promotes improved forelimb motor function and enhanced dendritic growth after focal ischemic injury. *Journal of Neuroscience, 21,* 5272–5280.

Author/Year	Study Objectives	Level/Design/Participants	Intervention & Outcome Measures	Results	Limitations
Brown et al. (2004)	Compare effects of stimulant treatment and motor experience on motor recovery	I—Randomized controlled trial $N = 48$ Sprague-Dawley rats; 5–8 per group	Researchers trained rats for 2 days in beam walking. Researchers then induced true lesion in rats that would constitute experimental groups, and sham lesions in the control group. They randomly assigned lesioned rats to lesion only, lesion training (one 2-hour session), lesion-amphetamine, lesion-amphetamine-training, lesion-limited experience, or lesion-amphetamine-limited experience group.	Training maximally enhanced motor recovery, amphetamine treatment delayed it, and limited experience affected it most negatively.	Study is of good quality.

Groups were tested 1 time per day for 10 days, except for 2 limited-experience groups that were tested on days 1 and 10 only.

Outcome:
• Beam walking

Reference: Brown, A. W., Bjelke, B., & Fuxe, K. (2004). Motor response to amphetamine treatment, task-specific training, and limited motor experience in a postacute animal stroke model. *Experimental Neurology, 190,* 102–108.

| Friel et al. (2000) | Determine if restriction of unimpaired hand was sufficient to retain spared (undamaged) hand area after injury or if retention of spared area required repetitive use of impaired hand | II—Nonrandomized controlled trial

N = 9 squirrel monkeys; 3 per group | Researchers assigned monkeys to restraint-training, restraint-no training, or no intervention. They trained restraint-training group to retrieve pellets with dominant hand from progressively smaller wells. Training occurred in 30-minute sessions 2 times per day 7 days per week until monkeys met criterion. Researchers then induced lesions in hand representational area of primary motor cortex of all three groups. Afterward, they restrained unimpaired hand of monkeys in restraint-training group, then again trained monkeys in pellet-retrieval task with impaired (dominant) hand until monkeys met criterion. Researchers also restrained unimpaired hand of monkeys in restraint-no training group but did not train monkeys. No-intervention group received no experience following lesion.

Outcomes:
• Motor skill (random probe trials on Klüver board)
• Changes in hand, digit, and wrist/forearm representational areas of primary motor cortex (electrophysiological mapping) | All groups showed significantly decreased motor skills during week 1 following lesion. All groups showed normal motor skills by 4 weeks following lesion.

At 1 month following lesion, restraint-training group showed significantly greater spared hand area than both other groups. Also, restraint-training group showed significantly greater spared digit area than no-intervention group, and restraint-training group tended to show greater total spared digit area than restraint-no training group. | The study had a small sample size; possible insensitivity of motor skill measure to subtle differences in behavior; possible effects of training before lesion, in restraint training group; and possibility of lesions not being large enough to allow differentiation of effects of various interventions. |

Reference: Friel, K. M., Heddings, A. A., & Nudo, R. J. (2000). Effects of postlesion experience on behavioral recovery and neurophysiologic reorganization after cortical injury in primates. *Neurorehabilitation and Neural Repair, 14,* 187–198.

(continued)

Evidence Table on Central Nervous System Plasticity: Animal Studies (continued)

Author/Year	Study Objectives	Level/Design/Participants	Intervention & Outcome Measures	Results	Limitations
Johansson (1996)	Investigate effects of housing rats in enriched environment after focal brain ischemia when transfer is delayed for 15 days following ischemia	II—Nonrandomized controlled trial $N = 15$ rats; 7 in enriched environment group, 8 in standard environment group	Researcher induced focal brain ischemia in rats and housed them in standard cages for 15 days. He then transferred 7 rats to enriched environment (larger cage containing various objects such as shelves, swings, etc.; objects changed weekly) for 7 weeks. Outcomes: • Ability to traverse rotating pole • Prehensile traction • Postural reflexes • Limb placement	Rats in enriched environment performed significantly better than rats in standard environment on traversing of pole, prehensile traction, and limb placement.	Lack of randomization

Reference: Johansson, B. B. (1996). Functional outcome in rats transferred to an enriched environment 15 days after focal brain ischemia. *Stroke, 27,* 324–326.

Author/Year	Study Objectives	Level/Design/Participants	Intervention & Outcome Measures	Results	Limitations
Humm et al. (1998)	Determine whether the brain is more susceptible to damaging loss in neural function associated with intense motor demands during the first week after injury as compared to during the second post-operative week	I—Randomized controlled trial $N = 54$ laboratory rats; randomly assigned to 7 groups	Random assignment to 7 groups Groups 1–4 ($n = 33$) received unilateral lesions to the forelimb representation area of the sensorimotor cortex. Sham animals in Groups 5–7 ($n = 21$) were anesthetized, but no lesion was made. Subgroups varied with regard to casting of the forelimb ipsilateral to the surgery, which forced the rats to rely on the impaired limb for postural support and movement. Groups 1 and 5 had no cast. Groups 2 and 6 were casted immediately after surgery for 1 week (early cast). Groups 3 and 7 were casted 8 days after surgery and wore the cast for 1 week (late cast). Group 4 was casted immediately after the surgery and wore the cast for 2 weeks (15-day cast).	Tissue volume: As expected, all lesioned animals had a significantly lower volume of remaining brain tissue as compared to sham-operated animals. Among lesion groups, there were significant differences between early-cast and no-cast animals ($p = 0.0001$) and between 15-day cast and no-cast animals ($p = 0.0001$). There was no significant difference ($p > 0.05$) in brain volume between rats in the early- and 15-day cast groups. Rats in the late-cast group had a significantly higher volume of remaining tissue when compared to the early-cast group, and there was no significant difference in brain volume between the late-cast and no-cast animals ($p > 0.05$).	Casts on the intact limb prevented the rat from using that forelimb for all normal behaviors rather than restricting to those activities requiring reaching and retrieval.

			Limb use asymmetry: All casted, lesioned groups showed significantly greater use of the impaired forelimb for landing from the rear position, but only on specific days. The authors interpreted results of videotape analysis to indicate that animals with restricted forelimb use showed poorer functional recovery than animals who were not casted.	
			From days 19–40, symmetry of forearm use (when landing on forelimbs from a rearing position) was observed.	
			On postsurgical day 40, all rats were sacrificed and lesion volume was measured.	

Reference: Humm, J. L., Kozlowski, D. A., James, D. C., Gotts, J. E., & Schallert, T. (1998). Use-dependent exacerbation of brain damage occurs during an early post-lesion vulnerable period. *Brain Research, 783*, 286–292.

| Jones et al. (1999) | Assess effects of training in complex motor skills on synaptic changes in layer V of opposite motor cortex, following unilateral lesion to forelimb representation area of sensorimotor cortex | I—Randomized controlled trial

N = 40 Long-Evans rats; 11 in lesion-and-training group, 9 in lesion-and-repetitive-exercise group, 10 in sham-and-training group, 10 in sham-and-repetitive-exercise group | Researchers induced lesions or performed sham operations on rats, then randomly assigned them to lesion and training, lesion and repetitive exercise, sham operation and training, or sham operation and repetitive exercise. Training focused on an acrobatic task. Repetitive exercise involved running back and forth in alley. Light training occurred for 1 trial per day on days 2–4 following surgery. Full training occurred for 4 trials per day on days 5–13, and 2 trials per day on days 14–28. Repetitive exercise occurred simultaneously and followed same pattern.

Outcomes:
• Synaptic changes in motor cortex
• Asymmetries in use of forelimb for postural support
• Sensorimotor function (Simultaneous Bilateral Tactile Stimulation Test; foot-fault test) | Lesion-and-repetitive-exercise rats showed significantly more layer V synapses per neuron than sham-and-repetitive-exercise rats. Sham-and-training rats showed significantly more synapses than sham-and-repetitive-exercise rats. Lesion-and-training rats showed significantly more synapses than sham-and-training rats or lesion-and-repetitive-exercise rats.

Lesion-and-training rats made significantly more errors in contralateral forelimb placement than sham-and-training rats. Both lesion groups showed significant elevation of use of ipsilateral forelimb and reduction of use of contralateral forelimb compared with both sham groups.

Lesion-and-training rats made significantly fewer foot-faults with both forelimbs than lesion-and-repetitive-exercise | Study is of good quality. |

(continued)

Evidence Table on Central Nervous System Plasticity: Animal Studies (continued)

Author/Year	Study Objectives	Level/Design/Participants	Intervention & Outcome Measures	Results	Limitations
				rats. Sham-and-training rats made significantly fewer foot-faults with both forelimbs than sham-and-repetitive-exercise rats. Both lesion groups made significantly more errors with the contralateral forelimb than the sham group of the same training condition.	

Reference: Jones, T. A., Chu, C. J., Grande, L. A., & Gregory, A. D. (1999). Motor skills training enhances lesion-induced structural plasticity in the motor cortex of adult rats. *Journal of Neuroscience, 19,* 10153–10163.

Author/Year	Study Objectives	Level/Design/Participants	Intervention & Outcome Measures	Results	Limitations
Leasure & Schallert (2004)	Investigate effects of complete disuse of impaired forelimb on later overuse of same limb	II—Nonrandomized controlled trial *N* = 89 Long-Evans rats; lesioned, 9–10 per group; sham, 5 per group	Researchers performed lesions or sham operations on rats, then assigned the rats to one of the following groups: 2 weeks disuse/1 week overuse, 1 week disuse/1 week overuse, and 1 week early disuse (all accomplished by casting contralateral limb); 1 week early overuse, 1 week late overuse (both accomplished by casting ipsilateral limb); and no casting (control).	On all outcome measurements except percent use of both limbs simultaneously for landing, sham-operated groups showed no significant differences among themselves, so researchers pooled data on them. On forelimb placing, all but one lesioned group (2 weeks disuse/1 week overuse) showed no significant differences from lesioned control, so researchers pooled data on them.	Possible bias from housing of rats in enriched environment

Reference: Leasure, J. L., & Schallert, T. (2004). Consequences of forced disuse of the impaired forelimb after unilateral cortical injury. *Behavioral Brain Research, 150,* 83–91.

Nudo et al. (1996)	Track topographies of distal forelimb representations in primary motor cortex before and after behavioral training for task requiring skilled use of hand digits	I—Randomized controlled trial Part 1: *N* = 6 squirrel monkeys; 3 in behavioral training group, 3 in control group Part 2: *N* = 1 control group monkey	Part 1: Researchers randomly assigned monkeys to behavioral training group or control group. Behavioral training group received training in retrieval of pellet from wells of progressively narrower width. Task emphasized use of digits. Control group had no training. Training occurred in 30-minute sessions 2 times per day until monkeys reached criterion (11 days in case of 2 monkeys, 50 days in case of 1 monkey). Researchers mapped representation of movements in distal forelimb zone of primary motor cortex. Part 2: One control group monkey received training in turning key. Task emphasized use of forearm. Training occurred at monkey's discretion 24 hours per day until monkey reached criterion. Researchers mapped representation as above. Outcome: • Evoked-movement digit and wrist or forearm representation (electrophysiological mapping)	Part 1: Electrophysiological mapping showed that after training, monkeys' evoked-movement digit representations expanded, whereas their evoked-movement wrist/forearm representations contracted. Part 2: Electrophysiological mapping showed that after training, monkey's evoked-movement digit representations contracted, whereas its evoked-movement forearm representations expanded.	Authors' attempt to control for sources of variability within and across mapping procedures may be questionable.
Plautz et al. (2000)	Evaluate whether repetitive motor use produces reorganization of cortical movement representations in primary motor cortex	I—Randomized control trial *N* = 7 squirrel monkeys; 3 in behaioral training group, 4 in control group	Part 1: Researchers randomly assigned monkeys to behavioral training group or control group. Behavioral training group received training in retrieval of pellet from well large enough to accommodate entire hand. Task did not call for acquisition of motor skill. Control group had no training. Training occurred in 30-minute sessions 2 times per day until monkeys reached criterion (15 days in case of 1 monkey, 13 days in case of 1 monkey, and 16 days in case of 1 monkey). Researchers mapped	Part 1: Monkeys in behavioral training group acquired no new motor skills, and mapping showed no systematic changes in extent of distal forelimb movement representations following training. Part 2: Results were same as above.	Study is of good quality.

Reference: Nudo, R. J., Milliken, G. W., Jenkins, W. M., & Merzenich, M. M. (1996). Use-dependent alterations of movement representations in primary motor cortex of adult squirrel monkeys. *Journal of Neuroscience, 16,* 785–807.

(continued)

Evidence Table on Central Nervous System Plasticity: Animal Studies *(continued)*

Author/Year	Study Objectives	Level/Design/Participants	Intervention & Outcome Measures	Results	Limitations
			representations of movements in distal forelimb zone of primary motor cortex. Part 2: In 1 monkey from behavioral training group, researchers repeated above procedure 6 months after completion of Part 1. Monkey reached criterion in 13 days. Researchers then mapped representations as above. Outcome: • Evoked-movement digit and wrist/forearm representation (electrophysiological mapping)		

Reference: Plautz, E. J., Milliken, G. W., & Nudo, R. J. (2000). Effects of repetitive motor training on movement representations in adult squirrel monkeys: Role of use versus learning. *Neurobiology of Learning and Memory, 74,* 27–55.

Evidence Table on Occupational Therapy and Adults With Stroke: Human Studies

Author/Year	Study Objectives	Level/Design/Participants	Intervention & Outcome Measures	Results	Study Limitations	Implications for OT
Ada et al. (2005)	Evaluate the effectiveness of supportive devices to prevent subluxation, reposition the head of the humerus in the glenoid fossa, decrease pain, and increase function after stroke	I—Systematic review; randomized, quasi-randomized, and controlled trials included Four trials with 142 participants who met the criteria	Trials examined the effectiveness of supportive devices (slings and strapping). Outcomes: • Pain • Function • Contracture	While there is evidence that shoulder strapping delays the onset of pain, there was no evidence that pain decreased, function increased, or contracture formation delayed. There was also no evidence that the use of slings or wheelchair attachments resulted in positive outcomes.	Only 1 study examined the effectiveness of the use of a sling with stoke survivors.	There is insufficient evidence to support the effectiveness of conventional shoulder slings or wheelchair attachments in preventing and treating shoulder subluxation after stroke.

Reference: Ada, L., Foongchomcheay, A., & Canning, C. (2005). Supportive devices for preventing and treating subluxation of the shoulder after stroke. *Cochrane Database of Systematic Reviews,* Issue No. 1, Art. No. CD003863.

Aisen et al. (1997)	Test whether robot-aided practice of an impaired limb influences recovery in stroke patients with hemiplegia	II—Nonrandomized controlled trial $N = 20$ (11 men, 9 women); 10 per group Average age: 60.9 years	On basis of impairment, participants were stratified to robot-aided therapy or sham robot-aided therapy. Robot-aided therapy consisted of goal-directed, robot-assisted arm movement, with video providing visual and auditory feedback. Sham therapy consisted of weekly or biweekly contact with robot, active movement of robot arm, and observation of response on video monitor. Intervention, delivered by rehabilitation therapists and robot in rehabilitation hospital, occurred 4–5 hours per week for experimental group and weekly or biweekly for control group, from admission until discharge (average 9.5 weeks). Outcomes: • Functional performance FIM • Motor impairment (upper-extremity section of Fugl-Meyer Assessment [FMA])	There were no significant differences between groups in scores on FIM, FMA, or distal MSS. The experimental group improved significantly more than control group on proximal MSS.	Lack of randomization and small sample size	Robot-aided therapy may provide new strategies to improve proximal arm motor function after stroke.

(continued)

Evidence Table on Occupational Therapy and Adults With Stroke: Human Studies *(continued)*

Author/Year	Study Objectives	Level/Design/Participants	Intervention & Outcome Measures	Results	Study Limitations	Implications for OT
			• Motor control and proportion of isolated volitional muscle activity involved in each movement (motor status scale [MSSI]) • Motor power (MP; assessment of power in biceps, triceps, and anterior and lateral deltoid muscles)			

Reference: Aisen, M. L., Krebs, H. I., Hogan, N., McDowell, F., & Volpe, B. T. (1997). The effect of robot-assisted therapy and rehabilitative training on motor recovery following stroke. *Archives of Neurology, 54,* 443–446.

Author/Year	Study Objectives	Level/Design/Participants	Intervention & Outcome Measures	Results	Study Limitations	Implications for OT
Barreca et al. (2003)	Review studies of treatment interventions for paretic upper limb of stroke patients	I—Systematic review of 68 studies (33 randomized controlled trials, 29 cohort studies, and 6 systematic reviews), followed by meta-analyses by type of intervention	Researchers identified 68 studies for review. They then conducted meta-analyses by type of intervention: exercise treatment; sensorimotor training; electrical stimulation alone, biofeedback alone, or a combination; electrical stimulation to prevent and treat shoulder pain and subluxation; movement and elevation to reduce hand edema; strapping of hemiplegic shoulder; and imagery.	Exercise treatment: Home exercises, repetitive training, and constraint-induced movement therapy had significant positive effects. Sensorimotor training: Stroke survivors receiving sensorimotor training improved significantly more than control groups. Electrical stimulation alone, biofeedback alone, or a combination: Stroke patients receiving electrical stimulation alone, or in combination with biofeedback, showed significantly more voluntary motor control of hemiplegic wrist and forearm than control groups. Electrical stimulation to prevent and treat shoulder pain and subluxation: Stroke patients receiving electrical stimulation showed a more significant decrease in glenohumeral subluxation than control groups.	Study is of good quality.	Sensorimotor training; motor learning training that includes use of imagery, electrical stimulation alone, or a combination of electrical stimulation and biofeedback; and engagement of the patient in repetitive, novel tasks can reduce motor impairment after stroke. Two treatment principles emerged from consensus exercise following review: If poor motor recovery is anticipated, treatment should focus on achieving and maintaining a comfortable, mobile arm and hand. If a higher degree of recovery is anticipated, treatment should focus on regaining function in upper limb.

Reference: Barreca, S., Wolf, S. L., Fasoli, S., & Bohannon, R. (2003). Treatment interventions for the paretic upper limb of stroke survivors: A critical review. *Neurorehabilitation and Neural Repair, 17,* 220–226.

Movement and elevation to reduce hand edema: Stroke patients who received a combination of movement and elevation showed significantly more improvement than control group that received elevation alone.

Strapping of hemiplegic shoulder: Stroke patients whose shoulders were strapped with Fixomull Stretch or Elastroplast Sports tape experienced significant decrease in pain compared with the control group.

Imagery: Stroke patients who viewed tape-recorded imagery and received conventional occupational therapy experienced significant reduction in motor impairment compared with control groups.

Bode et al. (2004)	Evaluate relative importance of therapy focus, therapy intensity, and length of stay to greater-than-expected functional gain, controlling for severity of stroke	II—Cohort design *N* = 198 (113 men, 85 women) Average age: 68.6 years	Researchers measured stroke severity at admission; self-care, mobility, and cognitive status at admission and discharge; therapy intensity by discipline and type of activity (function focused or impairment focused); length of stay; and residual change scores (difference between actual and predicted discharge status). Therapy, delivered by occupational therapists, physical therapists, and speech-language pathologists in 8 acute and 5 subacute facilities, occurred for average of 24.2 days. Occupational therapists delivered average of 3.46 15-minute units per day; physical therapists, 4.10 15-minute units per day; and speech-language	Controlling for severity, longer lengths of stay and more intensive function-focused occupational therapy predicted greater-than-expected gains in self-care and mobility. Longer lengths of stay alone predicted greater-than-expected cognitive gains.	Self-selection and the fact that lengths of stay during study were longer than they currently are may have caused bias; classification may not have produced information as useful as theoretically derived taxonomy would have produced. Therapies accounted for a significant proportion of variance in residual functional change. Both content and amount of therapy may be important in producing positive functional outcomes.

(continued)

Evidence Table on Occupational Therapy and Adults With Stroke: Human Studies *(continued)*

Author/Year	Study Objectives	Level/Design/Participants	Intervention & Outcome Measures	Results	Study Limitations	Implications for OT
			pathologists, 1.84 15-minute units per day. Outcomes: • Self-care • Mobility • Cognitive status • Gender • Length of stay • Function-focused intensity • Impairment-focused intensity			

Reference: Bode, R. K., Heinemann, A. W., Semik, P., & Mallinson, T. (2004). Relative importance of rehabilitation therapy characteristics on functional outcomes for persons with stroke. *Stroke, 35,* 2537–2542.

Author/Year	Study Objectives	Level/Design/Participants	Intervention & Outcome Measures	Results	Study Limitations	Implications for OT
Bowen et al. (2002)	Review studies of effects of cognitive rehabilitation on spatial neglect in stroke patients	I—Systematic review of 15 studies (8 randomized controlled trials, 7 nonrandomized controlled trials) *N* = 400 participants across 15 studies	Researchers reviewed controlled trials of cognitive rehabilitation for spatial neglect in stroke patients. Outcomes: • Scanning and attention skills (performance on standardized tests and assessments calling for target cancellation, line bisection, attention, and figure copying) • Functional recovery (independence in ADLs; Barthel Index and FIM) • Discharge destination (home or other)	Cognitive rehabilitation significantly improved experimental groups' scanning and attention skills as measured by cancellation and line-bisection tests compared with control groups. On functional recovery and discharge destination, however, there were no significant differences between experimental and control groups.	The studies reviewed had small sample sizes and poorly matched groups; the outcome measure (paper-and-pencil tests) most frequently used in studies reviewed was of questionable validity; many different interventions were used in the studies reviewed.	Cognitive rehabilitation seems to improve stroke patients' ability to complete tests—for example, canceling letters and bisecting lines. However, its effects on patients' ability to carry out meaningful daily tasks and live independently are not clear.

Reference: Bowen, A., Lincoln, N. B., & Dewey, M. (2002). Cognitive rehabilitation for spatial neglect following stroke. *Cochrane Database of Systematic Reviews,* Issue No. 2, Art. No. CD003586.

| Brogardh & Sjölund (2006) | Investigate effectiveness of 6 hours of constraint-induced group therapy wearing mitt on unaffected hand and investigate added benefits of use of mitt beyond therapy | III and I—Combined case-control and randomized controlled trial, respectively

$N = 16$ (9 men, 7 women); 9 in active-treatment group, 7 in control group

Average age: 56.7 years | All participants had had a stroke at least 6 months earlier. They agreed to use a mitt on the less affected hand 90% of waking hours for 12 consecutive days. They received constraint-induced movement therapy in small groups of 2–3 people 6 hours per day 5 times per week for 2 weeks. Therapy was delivered by occupational therapists, physical therapists, and nurses. Participants then were assigned randomly to receive active treatment or no further treatment (control). The active-treatment group used the mitt at home 90% of waking hours every other day for 2 weeks during 3 months—a total of 21 days. The control group stopped use of the mitt after group therapy but was encouraged to use affected hand in real-life situations.

Outcomes:
• Quality of movement and speed of performance (modified Motor Assessment Scale)
• Ability to grasp different objects (Sollerman Hand Function Test)
• Sensory discrimination (Two-Point Discrimination Test)
• Quality and amount of movement (Motor Activity Log [MAL]) | During constraint-induced group therapy, 11 of 16 participants significantly improved quality and speed of movement, and 12 of 16 improved the ability to grasp. Changes in self-reported quality and amount of use (MAL) also were significant.

After 3 months of extended use of the mitt, the active-treatment group showed no further significant improvement. The control group also showed no further significant improvement. | The first phase of study lacked a control group; small sample size; possible bias from the failure of some members of the active-treatment group to comply fully with extended wearing of the mitt. | Conducting constraint-induced movement therapy in small groups (2–3 patients per therapist) may be a realistic alternative to one-on-one treatment of stroke patients. |

Reference: Brogardh, C., & Sjölund, B. H. (2006). Constraint-induced movement therapy in patients with stroke: A pilot study on effects of small group training and of extended mitt use. *Clinical Rehabilitation, 20,* 218–227.

(continued)

Evidence Table on Occupational Therapy and Adults With Stroke: Human Studies (continued)

Author/Year	Study Objectives	Level/Design/Participants	Intervention & Outcome Measures	Results	Study Limitations	Implications for OT
Corr & Bayer (1995)	Evaluate effectiveness of occupational therapy interventions with stroke patients after discharge from stroke unit	I—Randomized controlled trial $N = 110$ (41 men, 69 women); 55 per group Average age: 75.5 years	Participants were randomly assigned to the occupational therapy intervention group or control group. Occupational therapy intervention was based on the Model of Human Occupation and included teaching new skills, facilitating more independence in ADLs, facilitating return of function, enabling use of equipment supplied by other agencies, and providing information and referrals. The control group received no treatment. Intervention delivered by occupational therapist in participants' homes occurred at 2, 8, 16, and 24 weeks after discharge. Outcomes: • ADLs (Barthel Index, Nottingham Extended ADL Scale) • Psychosocial well-being (Geriatric Depression Scale) • Quality of life (Pearlman's Quality of Life Scale) • Environment (home circumstances, use of services, and aid provided) • Hospital readmission	At 1 year after discharge, the experimental group performed significantly better on only two items of Nottingham Extended ADL Scale: feeding and telephone use. The experimental group also received significantly more aids (not provided by occupational therapy) and had significantly fewer hospital readmissions.	There were a large number of dropouts; attention bias; possibility of too few interventions to be effective; too many outcomes were measured, some unrelated to treatment.	Providing occupational therapy interventions for stroke patients after hospital discharge may not be effective in enhancing patients' ADL, depression status, or quality of life. It is a potential service-delivery model, but research with higher intensity of treatment is needed to determine effectiveness.

Reference: Corr, S., & Bayer, A. (1995). Occupational therapy for stroke patients after hospital discharge—A randomized controlled trial. *Clinical Rehabilitation, 9,* 291–296.

| Dean & Shepherd (1997) | Evaluate effect of task-related training on stroke patients' performance of seated reaching tasks | I—Randomized controlled trial; before-and-after design

N = 20 (gender not reported); 10 per group

Average age: 67.6 years | The experimental group received training to improve sitting balance. Training involved emphasizing appropriate loading of affected leg while practicing reaching tasks using the unaffected hand. The control group received sham training involving performance of cognitive-manipulative tasks while seated at table. Training, delivered by physical therapist (first author) in participants' homes, took place in ten 30-minute sessions over 2 weeks.

Outcomes:
• Seated reaching ability, as reflected in maximum distance, speed, and ground reaction forces (GRF) through affected foot (videotape of participants using the unaffected hand to reach forward, 45° toward unaffected side [ipsilateral], and 45° toward affected side [across])
• Sit-to-stand ability (measurement of GRF)
• Walking speed (stopwatch)
• Cognitive function (letter-cancellation task, word-finding task, and mathematics questions) | On maximum reaching distance in all directions, speed in diagonal reaches, and peak GRF for forward and across reaches, the experimental group performed significantly better than the control group.

On sit-to-stand ability, the experimental group significantly increased peak vertical GRF from before training to after.

The control group performed significantly better than experimental group on letter-cancellation task. | Possible bias from experimenter's expectations | A short task-related training program can improve stroke patients' performance on seated reaching tasks to near normal. Training may generalize to biomechanically similar actions. |

Reference: Dean, C. M., & Shepherd, R. B. (1997). Task-related training improves performance of seated reaching tasks after stroke: A randomized controlled trial. Stroke, 28, 722–728.

(continued)

Evidence Table on Occupational Therapy and Adults With Stroke: Human Studies (continued)

Author/Year	Study Objectives	Level/Design/Participants	Intervention & Outcome Measures	Results	Study Limitations	Implications for OT
Dolecheck & Schkade (1999)	Compare effectiveness of personally meaningful, goal-directed therapeutic activities for stroke patients with the effectiveness of activities that are not personally meaningful, in facilitating improvement in dynamic standing endurance	II—Counterbalanced repeated-measures design $N = 7$ (4 men, 3 women) Average age: 61.7 years	Participants completed an interest questionnaire and checklist, then identified their most preferred activity for inclusion in treatment. Treatment sessions began alternately with meaningful or nonmeaningful activity (i.e., if first session began with meaningful activity, second session began with nonmeaningful one). The activity required standing and was observed by a data collector. Intervention, delivered by occupational therapist, occurred in 45-minute sessions 3 times per week for 4 weeks. Outcome: • Standing tolerance (length of time standing)	Participants stood significantly longer when performing meaningful tasks than when performing nonmeaningful ones.	Small sample size; possible bias from data collector's expectations; possible selection bias (participants who did meaningful activity first were younger and female).	Findings support the occupational therapy assumption that engagement in personally meaningful tasks results in greater therapeutic gains. Dynamic standing endurance may improve when persons with hemiplegia perform meaningful activities in the context of exercise to improve standing tolerance.

Reference: Dolecheck, J. R., & Schkade, J. K. (1999). The extent dynamic standing endurance is effected when CVA subjects perform personally meaningful activities rather than nonmeaningful tasks. *Occupational Therapy Journal of Research, 19,* 40–54.

Author/Year	Study Objectives	Level/Design/Participants	Intervention & Outcome Measures	Results	Study Limitations	Implications for OT
Donkervoort et al. (2001)	Evaluate the efficacy of strategy training for left hemisphere stroke survivors with apraxia	I—Randomized controlled trial $N = 113$ (56 strategy training, 57 usual treatment) Participants recruited from 49 Dutch institutions (rehabilitation centers and nursing homes) Inclusion criteria: Left hemisphere stroke, apraxia, inpatient care	Strategy training: Participants are taught internal and external strategies (e.g., self-verbalization) to compensate for apraxia during the performance of ADLs. Usual occupational therapy: Concentrates on (sensory) motor, cognitive, and perceptual deficits of the survivor of a stroke and focuses on increasing independent function in ADLs Outcomes: • After 8 week treatment period and after 5 months • ADL observations—based on the performance of 4 standardized tasks	Participants in the strategy training group improved significantly more on the ADL observations with a small to medium effect on ADL functioning. There also was a medium significant effect for improvement on the Barthel Index for the strategy training group. There were no differences between groups at 5 month follow-up. Participants in the usual occupational therapy group received significantly more occupational therapy during the follow-up period than the	ADL observations measure may have a ceiling effect that could mask the effects of the strategy training group.	Strategy training is an effective intervention for improving ADL skills in stroke survivors with apraxia.

			Outcome Measures	Intervention	Results	Limitations	Conclusion
			• Barthel Index • Extended ADL judgment list filled in by occupational therapist and patient based on Rivermead Activities of Daily Living Scale • Apraxia Test • Motricity Index measures voluntary movement on affected side Questionnaire of therapies (e.g., occupational, physical) received during study period		strategy training period. This may have indicated that those in usual care may have required more occupational therapy to achieve the same outcome as strategy training group.		

Reference: Donkervoort, M., Dekker, J., Stehmann-Saris, F. C., & Deelman, B. G. (2001). Effect of strategy training in left hemisphere stroke patients with apraxia: A randomized clinical trial. *Neuropsychological Rehabilitation, 11,* 549–566.

Author/Year	Objective	Level/Design	Intervention	Results	Limitations	Conclusion
Drummond & Walker (1995, 1996)	Examine whether a leisure rehabilitation "program would encourage stroke patients to participate in leisure activities	I—Randomized controlled trial *N* = 65 (37 men, 28 women); 21 in leisure rehabilitation group, 21 in conventional occupational therapy group, and 23 in control group Average age: 65.9 years	Participants were randomly assigned to leisure rehabilitation group, conventional occupational therapy group, or control group (no leisure or occupational therapy). The leisure rehabilitation group received treatment needed for leisure pursuits; provision of equipment; advice on obtaining financial assistance and transport; liaison with specialist organizations; and provision of physical assistance, such as referral to voluntary agencies. The conventional occupational therapy group participated in traditional activities, such as transfers and dressing practice. It received no help or advice regarding leisure pursuits. Interventions, delivered by occupational therapist in participants' homes, took place in 30-minute sessions 1 time per week for 3 months, then every other week for 3 months.	The leisure rehabilitation group showed a significant increase in leisure scores at both 3 and 6 months after discharge. It also performed significantly better than other two groups on some items of Nottingham Extended ADL Scale (mobility at 3 and 6 months, leisure at 6 months) and Nottingham Health Profile (energy at 3 months, mobility at 3 and 6 months).	Possible bias from therapist's expectations; possible sampling bias (leisure rehabilitation group was younger)	A leisure rehabilitation program may be effective in enhancing stroke patients' leisure participation, as well as mobility and psychological well-being.

(continued)

Author/Year	Study Objectives	Level/Design/Participants	Intervention & Outcome Measures	Results	Study Limitations	Implications for OT
			Outcomes: • Leisure activities (Nottingham Leisure Questionnaire) • ADLs (Nottingham Extended ADL Scale) • Psychological well-being (Nottingham Health Profile) • Depression (Wakefield Depression Inventory)			

References: Drummond, A. E. R., & Walker, M. F. (1995). A randomized controlled trial of leisure rehabilitation after stroke. *Clinical Rehabilitation, 9,* 283–290.

Drummond, A. E. R., & Walker, M. F. (1996). Generalisation of the effects of leisure rehabilitation for stroke patients. *British Journal of Occupational Therapy, 59,* 330–334.

Author/Year	Study Objectives	Level/Design/Participants	Intervention & Outcome Measures	Results	Study Limitations	Implications for OT
Fasoli et al. (2003)	Examine effects of robotic therapy on motor impairment and recovery of function in hemiparetic arm of stroke patients	I—Randomized controlled trial *N* = 20 (16 men, 4 women); 13 in sensorimotor-exercise group, 7 in progressive-resistive-exercise group Average age: 55.5 years	Participants were assigned to robotic therapy involving either sensorimotor exercise or progressive resistive exercise. Intervention, delivered in rehabilitation hospital, occurred in 1-hour sessions 3 times per week for 6 weeks. Outcomes: • Muscle spasticity (Modified Ashworth Scale) • Presence of synergistic and isolated movement patterns and grasp (upper extremity section of Fugl-Meyer Assessment) • Motor power (Medical Research Council score) • Upper limb isolated movement and motor function—shoulder and elbow, and wrist and finger (Motor Status Scale)	Both groups improved significantly on three of four outcome measures. The progressive-resistive-exercise group showed significantly more improvement in wrist and hand movement than the sensorimotor-exercise group.	Possible bias from the method of assignment (participants in progressive-resistive-exercise group experienced different durations of training) and small sample size	Intensive robotic therapy may complement other approaches by decreasing chronic motor impairments in stroke patients with moderate to severe upper limb dysfunction.

Reference: Fasoli, S. E., Krebs, H. I., Stein, J., Frontera, W. R., & Hogan, N. (2003). Effects of robotic therapy on motor impairment and recovery in chronic stroke. *Archives of Physical Medicine and Rehabilitation, 84,* 477–482.

Author (Year)	Study Objectives	Level/Design/Participants	Intervention and Outcome Measures	Results	Study Limitations	Implications for Occupational Therapy
Fasoli et al. (2002)	Examine effects of verbal instructions on movement organization in stroke patients and persons without disability	I—Randomized controlled trial; counterbalanced repeated-measures design $N = 33$ (14 men, 19 women); 16 with stroke, 17 without disability (control group) Average age: Not reported	Participants were randomly assigned to receive externally focused instructions first or internally focused instructions first as they performed three tasks. Externally focused instructions addressed task-related parameters (e.g., location, size, or weight of object to be lifted); internally focused instructions addressed internal-movement factors (e.g., actual movements of elbow, wrist, or fingers). Three differet tasks were presented in random order. Participants performed 8 trials under each task-condition combination. Outcomes: • Movement time—speed (interval from beginning to end of reach) • Peak velocity—force (maximal instantaneous velocity associated with given movement) • Movement units (one acceleration phase and one deceleration phase) • Percentage of time to peak velocity (indicative of type of strategy selected, preplanned or guided)	For both groups, when instructions were externally focused, arm movements were significantly faster and more forceful than when internally focused.	Study is of good quality.	Stroke patients may benefit from instructions that focus on task-related parameters rather than on specific movement-related parameters.

Reference: Fasoli, S. E., Trombly, C. A., Tickle-Degnen, L., & Verfaellie, M. H. (2002). Effect of instructions on functional reach in persons with and without cerebrovascular accident. *American Journal of Occupational Therapy, 56,* 380–390.

(continued)

Evidence Table on Occupational Therapy and Adults With Stroke: Human Studies (continued)

Author/Year	Study Objectives	Level/Design/Participants	Intervention & Outcome Measures	Results	Study Limitations	Implications for OT
Fischer et al. (2004)	Examine relationship of self-awareness, goal-setting ability, and rehabilitation outcome in patients with brain injuries (stroke included)	III—Cross-sectional design $N = 63$ (32 men, 31 women); 45 with stroke, 10 with traumatic brain injury, 4 with multiple sclerosis, 3 with infection, and 1 with hypoxia Average age: 56.1 years	This was an observational study, with no intervention provided. Outcomes: • Awareness (clinicians' judgment and patient–clinician discrepancy on Patient Competency Rating Scale) • Goal-setting ability (self-set goals in experimental laboratory task; self-set goals for rehabilitation versus compentency rating by staff at discharge)	Patients' ratings of their awareness were significantly higher than clinicians' ratings on average. Patients' performance on the laboratory task was 10.2% lower than self-set goals, on average. Patients' goals for their rehabilitation outcome were 10.2% higher than staff's rating on average. Awareness measures predicted 32% of variance for goal-setting ability in rehabilitation context, but only 4% in cognitive task. Awareness measures predicted 33% of variance for rehabilitation outcome, but only 5% of variance for performance in cognitive task.	This study used mixed etiologies.	Awareness deficits in patients with brain injuries may be related to lower rehabilitation outcomes. Both variables may be connected to less realistic goal setting.

Reference: Fischer, S., Gauggel, S., & Trexler, L. E. (2004). Awareness of activity limitations, goal setting, and rehabilitation outcome in patients with brain injuries. Brain Injury, 18, 547–562.

Flinn et al. (2005)	Investigate the outcome of constraint-induced movement therapy (CIMT) on arm use, coordination, and perceptions of participation in meaningful activities	III—Before-and-after design $N = 11$ participants at least 6 months poststroke (7 males, 4 females) Average age: 61.4 years	Participants took part in a constraint-induced movement therapy program for 8 hours per day for 8 days, receiving therapy for 3.5 hours per day. The therapy included participation in activities with the affected hand and arm. Logs were kept during therapy and at home and included records of how long participants wore mitts on their unaffected arm. Outcomes: • MAL • Wolf Motor Function Test (WMFT) • COPM	Following treatment, participants significantly increased the use of their affected arm in daily activities as measured by the MAL. Coordination of the affected arm did not change as measured by the WMFT. While there was no change in satisfaction immediately following treatment, there was significant improvement in satisfaction with performance of activities at 4–6 months posttreatment as measured by the COPM. Participants did not identify improvements in occupational performance or	Small sample size, lack of a control group. The authors report that the social component of the program may have contributed to the positive improvements in performance.	CIMT is effective in increasing the use of the affected arm in daily activities and may increase satisfaction in the performance of occupations that require the use of the hand.

satisfaction as an outcome of CIMT.

Reference: Flinn, N. A., Schamburg, S., Fetrow, J. M., & Flanigan, J. (2005). The effect of constraint-induced movement treatment on occupational performance and satisfaction in stroke survivors. *OTJR: Occupation, Participation and Health, 25,* 119–127.

Author/Year	Objective	Design/Participants	Intervention/Outcomes	Results	Limitations	Implications
French et al. (2007)	Determine whether repetitive task training following stroke affects upper, lower, or global limb function. Examine whether treatment effects are dependent on qualities of practice.	I—Systematic review 14 randomized and quasi-randomized controlled trials were included in the review, with a total of 695 participants.	Interventions included in the review incorporated an active motor sequence performed repetitively within a single training session, had a functional goal, and measured the amount of practice. Outcomes: • Primary—Upper-limb function/ reach, lower-limb function/ reach, and global motor function • Secondary—ADLs, motor impairment, quality of life	The results of the review indicate that those in the repetitive-task training had significantly better walking distance, walking speed, sit-to-stand, and ADL function. There were no differences for quality of life, impairment measures, functional ambulation, and global motor function. No differences were noted on any measure were noted at 6- or 12-month follow-up.	Heterogeneity of populations included in review and studies were limited to those less than 6 months poststroke.	Repetitive tasks training is indicated for improving motor function related to walking, sit to stand, and ADL function in stroke survivors.

Reference: French, B., Thomas, L. H., Leathley, M. J., Sutton, C. J., McAdam, J., Forster, A., et al. (2007). Repetitive task training for improving functional ability after stroke. *Cochrane Database of Systematic Reviews,* Issue No. 4, Art. No. CD006073.

Author/Year	Objective	Design/Participants	Intervention/Outcomes	Results	Limitations	Implications
Fritz et al. (2006)	Investigate 6 potential predictors of outcomes of CIMT	III—Before-and-after design N = 55 (33 men, 22 women) Average age: 62.1 years	Participants received constraint-induced movement therapy involving task practice with the affected hand and arm. They wore a mitt on the unaffected hand for goal of 90% of waking hours. Therapy occurred 6 hours per day 5 days per week for 2 weeks. Potential predictors were side of stroke, time since stroke, hand dominance, age, sex, and ambulatory status. Outcomes: • Movement capability (performance-time scale of WMFT) • Amount of perceived use	Age was the only significant predictor of outcome at 4–6 months, and only for amount of perceived use.	Lack of randomization and possible bias from withdrawals	Age may be a significant predictor of favorable outcome from constraint-induced movement therapy. Side of stroke, time since stroke, hand dominance, sex, and ambulatory status were not predictors and therefore should not be considered as inclusion criteria in CIMT programs.

Reference: Fritz, S. L., Light, K. E., Clifford, S. N., Patterson, T. S., Behrman, A. L., & Davis, S. B. (2006). Descriptive characteristics as potential predictors of outcomes following constraint-induced movement therapy for people after stroke. *Physical Therapy, 86,* 825–832.

(continued)

Evidence Table on Occupational Therapy and Adults With Stroke: Human Studies *(continued)*

Author/Year	Study Objectives	Level/Design/Participants	Intervention & Outcome Measures	Results	Study Limitations	Implications for OT
Geusgens et al. (2006)	Evaluate the transfer effects of cognitive strategy training for stroke survivors with apraxia	III—Pretest/posttest *N* = 29 patients with left-hemisphere stroke; apraxia; and judgment made by attending physician, occupational therapist, and patient that apraxia should be treated Referrals from Dutch rehabilitation centers (14) and nursing homes (2)	From a list of 14 ADL tasks of similar level of difficulty, participants selected 6 that they wanted to relearn. Occupational therapists used a standardized cognitive strategy training developed by van Heugten and colleagues (1998) to teach patients to compensate for the presence of apraxia during an 8-week program. Examples of the strategies include verbalization and pictures showing the correct order of task performance. Outcomes: • ADL observations—based on the performance of 4 standardized tasks • Barthel Index • Evaluated performance on new tasks and in new situation (rehabilitation center versus home) • Evaluation at completion of training and 5 months after the start of training • Apraxia test • Functional Motor Test	Participants in the cognitive strategy training improved significantly for performance of trained and new tasks at the end of the 8-week program, which was retained at follow-up. There were also no significant differences between performance at the rehabilitation center and at home, indicating transfer of training effects.	Lack of control and loss to follow-up	Generalization to new tasks should be a goal of cognitive strategy training for stroke survivors who have apraxia.

Reference: Geusgens, J. A. V., van Heugten, C. M., Cooijmans, J. P. J., Jolles, J., & van den Heuvel, W. J. A. (2006). Transfer effects of a cognitive strategy training for stroke patients with apraxia. *Journal of Clinical and Experimental Neuropsychology, 29,* 831–841.

| Geusgens et al. (2007) | Evaluate the effectiveness of cognitive strategy training for persons with acquired brain injury (including stroke) | I—Systematic review

Review included electronic searches of PubMed, PsychInfom EMBASE, and CINAHL | All studies included were intervention studies of cognitive strategy training. This was defined as training to teach patients new ways to execute daily activities by using either internal or external strategies to compensate for cognitive impairments. | 39 papers describing 41 studies were included in the review. Cognitive strategy training was evaluated in seven domains of functioning: information processing, problem solving/executive functioning, memory/attention, language, neglect, apraxia, and daily activities. Most studies included in the review reported at least one type of transfer. | Methodological quality of included studies was low. Many included studies with small sample sizes. One-half of included studies were single-subject designs. Several studies with positive results did not statistically evaluate results of study, especially in those studies evaluating transfer to daily life. | There is research support for the capacity of stroke survivors to generalize learned cognitive strategies to new tasks that were never practiced during therapy sessions. However, more studies, with higher levels of methodological quality, are needed. |

Outcome:
- Evaluated transfer to non-trained items, standardized daily tasks, or daily life.

Reference: Geusgens, C. A. V., Winkens, I., van Heugten, C. M., Jolles, J., & van den Heuvel, W. J. A. (2007). Occurrence and measurement of transfer in cognitive rehabilitation: A critical review. *Journal of Rehabilitation Medicine, 39,* 425–439.

| Gibson & Schkade (1997) | Examine use of occupational adaptation (OA) frame of reference in evaluation and treatment of stroke patients | II—Cohort design

N = 50 (20 men, 30 women); 25 per group

Average age: 74 years | Stroke patients admitted to facility after implementation of OA served as the experimental group. They identified role and context, which became the focus of intervention, and regularly evaluated their own progress. Therapist targeted a combination of component abilities and performance skills.

Patients most recently discharged from a facility served as control group. They received standard evaluations and treatment. Occupational therapists delivered treatments in hospital daily until patients were discharged. Average length of stay of OA group was 2.12 weeks; control group, 3.28 weeks.

Outcomes:
• ADLs (facility-generated ADL scale)
• Environment (discharge environment) | Experimental group members achieved significantly higher levels of functional independence, and significantly more of them were discharged to less restrictive environments than control group members. | Use of cohort design, precluding establishment of causal relationship; possible bias from therapists' expectations | Client-centered approach may be effective in planning treatment and evaluating progress. Also, targeting a combination of component abilities and performance skills may be effective. |

Reference: Gibson, J. W., & Schkade, J. K. (1997). Occupational adaptation intervention with patients with cerebrovascular accident: A clinical study. *American Journal of Occupational Therapy, 51,* 523–529.

(continued)

Evidence Table on Occupational Therapy and Adults With Stroke: Human Studies (continued)

Author/Year	Study Objectives	Level/Design/Participants	Intervention & Outcome Measures	Results	Study Limitations	Implications for OT
Gilbertson et al. (2000)	Evaluate whether brief program of occupational therapy in home could improve recovery of stroke patients just discharged from hospital	I—Randomized controlled trial N = 138 (60 men, 78 women); 67 in experimental group, 71 in control group Average age: 71.0 years	Participants were randomly assigned to intervention service plus routine services, or routine services alone. Intervention service involved treatment tailored to recovery goals identified by participant (e.g., regaining self-care activities). Routine services involved multidisciplinary inpatient rehabilitation, provision of support services and equipment, regular multidisciplinary review at stroke clinic, and, for selected participants, predischarge home visit and referral to medical day hospital. Occupational therapists delivered intervention service in participants' homes. Treatment occurred in 30- to 45-minute sessions about 10 times over 6 weeks. Outcomes: • Extended ADLs (Nottingham Extended ADL Scale) • Global outcome of deterioration (Barthel Index or death) • Satisfaction with outpatient services (questionnaire) • Resource use (place of residence, hospital readmissions, provision of equipment and services, costs incurred by participants and caregivers, and staff time) • Health (measures of subjective health)	At 8 weeks, participants in intervention-plus-routine-services group had significantly higher performance on Nottingham Extended ADL Scale than those in routine-services-alone group, after adjustment for baseline Barthel Index. Also, those in intervention-plus-routine-services group had a significantly better global outcome than those in routine-services-alone group. Regarding satisfaction, participants in the intervention-plus-routine-services group were significantly more likely to agree that "things were well prepared for returning home" and they knew whom to contact with problems relating to their stroke. At 6 months, although, results on primary outcomes were no longer statistically significant. Groups were evenly matched on place of residence, hospital readmissions, equipment and services provided, and costs incurred	Possible bias from assessor's expectations and from method of follow-up at 6 months (via mail rather than by interview)	Findings support extending occupatioal therapy services into period following discharge from hospital after stroke.

Reference: Gilbertson, L., Langhorne, P., Walker, A., Allen, A., & Murray, G. D. (2000). Domiciliary occupational therapy for patients with stroke discharged from hospital: Randomised controlled trial. *British Medical Journal, 320,* 603–606.

Author/Year	Study Objectives	Level/Design and Participants	Intervention and Outcome Measures	Results	Study Limitations	Conclusions
Goldenberg et al. (2004)	Investigate effect of tactile feedback on pantomiming of tool use in stroke patients with apraxia	II—Nonrandomized controlled trial N = 10 participants (6 men, 4 women) Average age: 51.1 years	Participants were asked to demonstrate use of 12 tools with their impaired hand under three conditions: pantomime with visual input (photograph of tool), pantomime with visual and tactile input (photograph of tool and wooden implement resembling handle of tool), and real use (actual tool). Researchers counterbalanced presentation of conditions. Conditions were presented by experimenter. Outcomes: • Shaping of hand • Movement • Position of hand (All three outcomes were assessed by scorers viewing videotape of tests.)	Participants performed significantly better on all three outcome measures under real use than under either of other conditions. Participants did not perform significantly better under pantomime with visual and tactile input than under pantomime with visual input only; however, there was wide variation among individuals in reaction to tactile feedback, some showing considerable improvement and others showing considerable deterioration.	The study lacked randomization.	Real-tool use is preferable to pantomimed-tool use, even with tactile input, in improving motor performance.

Reference: Goldenberg, G., Hentze, S., & Hermsdörfer, J. (2004). The effect of tactile feedback on pantomime of tool use in apraxia. *Neurology, 63*, 1863–1867.

| Greenberg & Fowler (1980) | Compare effectiveness of kinesthetic biofeedback and traditional occupational therapy intervention on elbow range of motion in stroke patients | I—Randomized controlled trial

N = 20 (13 men, 7 women); 10 per group

Average age: 64.9 years | Participants were randomly assigned to kinesthetic biofeedback group or control group. The kinesthetic biofeedback group received audiovisual kinesthetic feedback on active elbow extension through electrogoniometer and shaping. The control group received conventional occupational therapy (Brunnstrom treatment). Interventions, delivered by an occupational therapist in hospital, occurred in 30-minute sessions 2 times per week for 4 weeks.

Outcome:
• Elbow range of motion (traditional goniometer) | There was no significant difference between groups. The majority of participants in each group achieved increase in active elbow extension. | Possible bias from experimenters' expectations | Kinesthetic biofeedback may be as effective in improving elbow active range of motion as conventional occupational therapy focusing on motor components. |

Reference: Greenberg, S., & Fowler, R. S., Jr. (1980). Kinesthetic biofeedback: A treatment modality for elbow range of motion in hemiplegia. *American Journal of Occupational Therapy, 34*, 738–743.

(continued)

Evidence Table on Occupational Therapy and Adults With Stroke: Human Studies (continued)

Author/Year	Study Objectives	Level/Design/Participants	Intervention & Outcome Measures	Results	Study Limitations	Implications for OT
Hsieh et al. (1996)	Compare the effects of added-purpose occupations and rote exercise on exercise repetitions in stroke patients with hemiplegia	I—Randomized controlled trial; counterbalanced repeated-measures design N = 21 (12 men, 9 women) Average age: 64.5 years	Participants were randomly assigned to one of three sequences for completion of three conditions: added-materials occupation, involving throwing small balls; imagery-based occupation, involving imagining themselves throwing small balls; and rote exercise, involving execution of same movements without materials or imagery. Participants were to do their best and stop when tired. Each participant completed each condition on separate days. All participants completed all conditions within 1 week. Interventions were delivered by occupational therapist in hospital. Outcomes: • Frequency of repetitions • Duration of repetitions • Frequency of discontinuities	Participants did significantly more repetitions in added-materials and imagery-based conditions than in rote-exercise condition.	Study is of good quality.	Use of materials that foster occupations or imagery may facilitate motor performance in stroke patients by increasing adherence to therapy routines.

Reference: Hsieh, C. L., Nelson, D. L., Smith, D. A., & Peterson, C. Q. (1996). A comparison of performance in added-purpose occupations and rote exercise for dynamic standing balance in persons with hemiplegia. *American Journal of Occupational Therapy, 50,* 10–16.

Author/Year	Study Objectives	Level/Design/Participants	Intervention & Outcome Measures	Results	Study Limitations	Implications for OT
Jongbloed & Morgan (1991)	Determine efficiency of occupational therapy intervention related to leisure activities of stroke survivors	I—Randomized controlled trial N = 40 (27 men, 13 women); 20 per group Average age: 69.6 years	Experimental group members received occupational therapy intervention aimed at helping them resume previous leisure activities, engage in new ones, or do both. Control group members were interviewed about involvement in leisure activities and about the effects of stroke on their lives. Intervention, delivered by occupational therapist in participants'	There were no significant differences between groups in amount of or satisfaction with involvement.	There may have been too few visits to evaluate effectiveness; possible bias from control group also being involved in leisure activities.	This study's findings do not promote support for effectiveness of occupational therapy interventions specifically aimed at restarting leisure activities after stroke.

homes, occurred in 1-hour sessions 1 time per week for 5 weeks.

Outcome:
- Leisure activities (subscales of Katz Adjustment Index re: amount of and satisfaction with activity involvement)

Reference: Jongbloed, L., & Morgan, D. (1991). An investigation of involvement in leisure activities after a stroke. *American Journal of Occupational Therapy, 45,* 420–427.

| Jongbloed et al. (1989) | Compare the effectiveness of two occupational therapy approaches in treating stroke patients | I—Randomized controlled trial

N = 90 (41 men, 49 women); 47 in functional treatment group, 43 in sensorimotor integrative approach group

Average age: 71.3 years | Participants were randomly assigned to the functional treatment group or the sensorimotor integrative group. Functional treatment involved teaching participants ADLs and instrumental activities of daily living (IADLs) tasks. A sensorimotor integrative approach involved treating sensorimotor deficits using neurodevelopmental interventions.

Interventions, delivered by occupational therapists in hospital, occurred in 40-minute sessions 5 days per week for 8 weeks.

Outcomes:
- ADLs (Barthel Index)
- Home maintenance (meal preparation)
- Sensorimotor integration (8 subtests of Sensorimotor Integration Test Battery) | Both groups improved significantly over time on all outcome measures except 3 of 8 sensorimotor integration subtests. There were no significant differences between groups on any outcome measures. | The study had no control group (which would have controlled for possibility of spontaneous recovery); possible equalization of treatment by co-intervention (both groups receiving similar assistance in self-care, medical and nursing care, and physical therapy). | Functional treatment may be as beneficial as sensorimotor integrative approach. |

Reference: Jongbloed, L., Stacey, S., & Brighton, C. (1989). Stroke rehabilitation: Sensorimotor integrative treatment versus functional treatment. *American Journal of Occupational Therapy, 43,* 391–397.

(continued)

Evidence Table on Occupational Therapy and Adults With Stroke: Human Studies (*continued*)

Author/Year	Study Objectives	Level/Design/Participants	Intervention & Outcome Measures	Results	Study Limitations	Implications for OT
Legg et al. (2006)	Determine whether occupational therapy focused on personal ADLs improves recovery following stroke	I—Systematic review of 10 studies (all randomized controlled trials) N = 1,348 over 10 studies	Researchers reviewed randomized controlled trials of occupational therapy intervention in which stroke patients practiced personal ADLs or stroke patients' performance of ADLs was the focus, versus usual care or no care. Outcomes: • Performance of personal ADLs • Death or poor outcome (having deteriorated, being dependent, or requiring institutional care)	Stroke patients who had received occupational therapy intervention were less likely to deteriorate and more likely to be independent in performance of personal ADLs. Exact nature of the intervention to achieve maximum benefit (what should be provided, when, how often, etc.) is highly individualized.	Possible bias in trials reviewed, from therapists' expectations, contamination (provision of intervention to control group), and co-intervention (same therapist providing additional care to treatment or control group).	Occupational therapy interventions reduce stroke patients' chances of deterioration in performance of ADLs and benefit patients in performance of personal and extended ADLs.

Reference: Legg, L. A., Drummond, A. E., & Langhorne, P. (2006). Occupational therapy for patients with problems in activities of daily living after stroke. *Cochrane Database of Systematic Reviews,* Issue No. 4, Art. No. CD003585.

Author/Year	Study Objectives	Level/Design/Participants	Intervention & Outcome Measures	Results	Study Limitations	Implications for OT
Lenze et al. (2004)	Compare functional outcomes and length of stay in relation to stroke patients' levels of participation in physical and occupational therapy	II—Prospective observational study, cohort design 242 (88 men, 154 women); 38 with stroke, 204 with other impairments; 139 good participators, 53 occasional poor participators, and 50 frequent poor participators Average age: Not reported (range of average ages across three levels of participation, 70.4–72.2 years)	Occupational therapists delivered therapy in 1-hour sessions, 1 time per day; physical therapists delivered therapy 2 times per day (duration not reported). Therapists rated participants' level of participation (using Pittsburgh Rehabilitation Participation Scale). Researchers then categorized participation as good, occasional poor, or frequent poor. Researchers compared these levels with participants' performance on outcome measures. Outcomes: • Functional status (FIM) • Length of stay • Discharge destination	Those designated as good participators constituted 57% of sample; those designated as occasional-poor participators, 22%; and those designated as frequent-poor participators, 21%. The good group participated significantly more than either of other groups. Good- and occasional-poor participators improved significantly more on functional status than frequent-poor participators. Occasional-poor participators had significantly longer lengths of stay than good or frequent-poor participators.	Possible bias from therapists' observations of participation (reflecting other factors, such as patients' poor progression in therapy or poor quality of patient–therapist relationship); too few stroke patients in sample	Occupational therapy practitioners should be alert to poor participation in therapy because of its implications for functional outcomes.

Good participators were discharged to home at rate of 94.0%, compared with 85.7% for occasional-poor participators and 84.1% for frequent-poor participators.

Reference: Lenze, E. J., Munin, M. C., Quear, T., Dew, M. A., Rogers, J. C., Begley, A. E., et al. (2004). Significance of poor patient participation in physical and occupational therapy for functional outcome and length of stay. *Archives of Physical Medicine and Rehabilitation, 85,* 1599–1601.

| Liepert (2006) | Investigate excitability of motor cortex in stroke patients before and after CIMT | III—Before-and-after design

N = 12 (7 men, 5 women)

Average age: 59.5 years | Researchers used transcranial magnetic stimulation (TMS) and peripheral electrical stimulation to assess excitability of motor cortex in participants. Participants then received constraint-induced movement therapy 6 hours per day for 12 days. Afterward, researchers reassessed excitability of motor cortex.

Outcomes:
• Motor thresholds (MTs)
• Motor evoked potential (MEP) latency and central motor conduction time
• Duration of silent period obtained by TMS with stimulus intensity 50% above MT
• Intracortical inhibition (ICI)
• Intracortical facilitation
• Amount and quality of use
• Motor function (WMFT)
• Spasticity (MAS) | MEP amplitudes were significantly different after therapy. MEP size was significantly and inversely correlated with MT.

Before therapy, participants had significantly less ICI in the affected hemisphere than in the unaffected hemisphere. After therapy, mean ICI value remained almost identical in both hemispheres, but a significant difference in amount of ICI changes was evident. ICI changes were stronger in the affected hemisphere.

Participants significantly improved motor function following therapy, and significantly reduced spasticity. | Lack of control group and randomization | CIMT enhances motor function in patients in the chronic phase of stroke and also produces evidence of recordable motor cortex excitability. |

Reference: Liepert, J. (2006). Motor cortex excitability in stroke before and after constraint-induced movement therapy. *Cognitive and Behavioral Neurology, 19,* 41–47.

(continued)

Evidence Table on Occupational Therapy and Adults With Stroke: Human Studies (continued)

Author/Year	Study Objectives	Level/Design/Participants	Intervention & Outcome Measures	Results	Study Limitations	Implications for OT
Liepert et al. (2000)	Use CIMT as a model to assess therapy-induced plasticity in stroke patients	III—Before-and-after design $N = 13$ (10 men, 3 women) Average age: 56.7 years	Participants received CIMT for 12 days. They wore a splint on the nonparetic arm all 12 days for 90% of waking hours and were trained in use of paretic arm 6 hours per day for 8 days. Intervention was delivered in laboratory. Outcomes: • Arm use in 20 ADLs (MAL) • Changes in cortical output area (TMS)	Participants significantly improved arm use. Size of muscle output area in affected hemisphere was significantly enlarged (nearly double in size).	Lack of control group and randomization	CIMT may induce alteration in brain function and improvement in motor function.

Reference: Liepert, J., Bauder, H., Wolfgang, H. R., Miltner, W. H., Taub, E., & Weiller, C. (2000). Treatment-induced cortical reorganization after stroke in humans. *Stroke, 31,* 1210–1216.

Author/Year	Study Objectives	Level/Design/Participants	Intervention & Outcome Measures	Results	Study Limitations	Implications for OT
Liepert et al. (2004)	Study impact of lesion in central somatosensory system, lesion in cerebellum, and CMIT on excitability of motor cortex	IV—Single-subject design Part 1: $N = 3$ Part 2: $N = 6$ Part 3, study A: $N = 15$; study B: $N = 8$ (Gender not reported for any part) Average age: Not reported	Researchers studied participants in part 1 for interaction between central somatosensory lesions and excitability of motor cortex; participants in part 2 for interaction between cerebellar lesions and excitability of motor cortex; and participants in part 3, studies A and B, for effects of constraint-induced movement therapy on excitability of motor cortex. Latter intervention occurred 6 hours per day 5 days per week for 2 weeks. Outcomes: • Interaction between central somatosensory lesion and motor excitability (TMS) • Interaction between cerebellar lesion and motor excitability	Participants in part 1 showed loss of intracortical inhibition on the affected side. Participants in part 2 showed loss of intracortical facilitation in the primary motor cortex. Participants in part 3, study A, showed significant improvement in motor function and enlarged motor output area for the paretic hand following therapy. Four participants in part 3, study B, showed less intracortical inhibition after therapy, and 4 showed more. Difference in values of intracortical inhibition before and	Small sample size and a lack of control group and randomization	CIMT may induce changes in neural excitability, mainly in affected hemisphere.

Author/Year	Study Objectives	Level/Design/Participants	Intervention and Outcome Measures	Results	Study Limitations
			• Motor function (MAL) • Changes in cortical motor output area (TMS and functional magnetic resonance imaging [fMRI])	after therapy was significantly stronger in the affected hemisphere than in the nonaffected hemisphere. Also, motor thresholds were reduced after therapy.	

Reference: Liepert, J., Hamzei, F., & Weiller, C. (2004). Lesion-induced and training-induced brain reorganization. *Restorative Neurology and Neuroscience, 22,* 269–277.

Author/Year	Study Objectives	Level/Design/Participants	Intervention and Outcome Measures	Results	Study Limitations
Lin et al. (1996)	Compare relative efficacy of four conditions in reducing left neglect during line bisection	I—Randomized controlled trial; counterbalanced repeated-measures design *N* = 13 (12 men, 1 woman) Average age: 57.5 years	Participants were randomly assigned to one of four sequences of conditions under which they were to bisect line: ABCD, BCDA, CDAB, and DABC. Condition A represented no cueing; condition B, visual cueing; condition C, digit circling; and condition D, digit circling plus finger tracing. Participants performed 1 condition per day for 4 consecutive days. Under each condition, participants performed 21 trials. Occupational therapists delivered intervention in hospital. Outcome: • Perceptual processing (line bisection)	Under all three cueing conditions, participants performed significantly better than under no-cueing condition. Digit circling plus finger tracing produced greatest improvement over baseline.	Small sample size

Reference: Lin, K.-C., Cermak, S. A., Kinsbourne, M., & Trombly, C. A. (1996). Effects of left-sided movements on line bisection in unilateral neglect. *Journal of the International Neuropsychological Society, 2,* 404–411.

Even with small sample size, results suggest use of visuomotor cueing (digit circling plus finger tracing) to reduce left neglect.

(continued)

Evidence Table on Occupational Therapy and Adults With Stroke: Human Studies (continued)

Author/Year	Study Objectives	Level/Design/Participants	Intervention & Outcome Measures	Results	Study Limitations	Implications for OT
Lin et al. (2007)	Assess outcomes of modified constraint-induced movement therapy (mCIMT) on motor control characteristics during performance of functional reach-to-grasp task (as measured by motion analysis technology) and functional performance	I—Pre–post randomized controlled trial. *N* = 32 patients with stroke who meet motor criteria for participation in CIMT	Participants were randomly assigned to mCIMT or control (TR) groups. Participants in both groups received individualized, 2-hour occupational therapy sessions 5 times per week, for 3 weeks Therapy for mCIMT participants consisted of shaping and adaptive, repetitive task practice techniques, with 15 minutes of therapy time spent on reducing abnormal muscle tone when needed. In addition, they wore mitts on the less affected hand every weekday for 6 hours during a time of frequent arm use. TR group members received traditional rehabilitation at the same dosage. Outcomes: • Kinematic analysis of spatial and temporal movement efficiency and type of movement control when reaching forward to grasp a beverage can • MAL • FIM Outcomes were assessed immediately after the 3-week intervention.	Analysis of covariance revealed significantly greater improvements for the mCIMT group in temporal, spatial, and preplanning measures generated by kinematic analysis, but more so when performing the bilateral task. The mCIMT improvements on MAL and FIM were also significantly greater than the TR group.	No follow-up assessments were made to assess long-term effects. Study did not include objects of different sizes to detect treatment efficacy on grasping.	This study provides additional support for the efficacy of mCIMT during rehabilitation of stroke survivors who meet the motor criteria for CIMT participation.

Reference: Lin, K.-C., Wu, C. Y., Wei, T. H., Lee, C. Y., & Liu, J. S. (2007). Effects of modified constraint-induced movement therapy on reach-to-grasp movements and functional performance after chronic stroke: A randomized controlled study. *Clinical Rehabilitation, 21,* 1075–1086.

Study	Purpose	Design/Participants	Methods/Outcomes	Results	Comments	Conclusions
Lincoln et al. (1997)	Investigate effect of perceptual assessment followed by treatment addressing perceptual deficits on perceptual impairment in stroke patients	I—Randomized controlled trial $N = 315$ (185 men, 130 women); 176 in stroke-unit group, 139 in conventional-ward group Average age: 68.1 years	Participants were randomly assigned to the stroke unit or conventional ward. All participants underwent perceptual assessment on entry to study and at 3, 6, and 12 months after randomization to groups. Stroke group then received intensive rehabilitation adjusted to nature of perceptual deficits. Stroke unit, with 15 beds, was staffed by 3 physical therapists, 2 occupational therapists, 1 speech therapist, and 1 part-time clinical psychologist. Conventional wards, with 24 beds each, were staffed by 1 physical therapist and 1 occupational therapist per ward. Speech therapy and clinical psychology were available by referral. Outcomes: • Independence in ADLs (Barthel Index and Rivermead ADL and Extended ADL Scale) • Motor function (Rivermead Motor Assessment) • Perceptual impairment (Rey figure copy)	At 3, 6, and 12 months, stroke-unit group showed significantly less perceptual impairment than conventional-ward group. Stroke-unit group had significantly better functional outcomes than conventional-ward group. Main predictors of ADL outcome at 12 months were scores at entry on Barthel Index, Rivermead Motor Assessment, and Rey figure copy; and age and ward type.	Study is of good quality.	Perceptual impairment has important effect on ADL outcome. Rehabilitation provided in a designated stroke unit is more effective than rehabilitation provided in a conventional hospital unit in reducing perceptual impairments and improving ADL outcomes.

Reference: Lincoln, N. B., Drummond, A. E., & Berman, P. (1997). Perceptual impairment and its impact on rehabilitation outcomes. *Disability and Rehabilitation, 19*, 231–234.

Study	Purpose	Design/Participants	Methods/Outcomes	Results	Comments	Conclusions
Logan et al. (1997)	Compare routine provision of occupational therapy by local authority social service departments with enhanced experimental service	I—Randomized controlled trial $N = 111$ (56 men, 55 women); 53 in experimental group, 58 in control group Average age: 72.6 years	Participants were randomly assigned to enhanced service or routine service. Members of the enhanced-service group were seen and treated by one occupational therapist (first author of article). Caseload was expected to be manageable enough that occupational therapist could see participants sooner than possible under routine service. Members of the routine-service group were prioritized by senior occupational therapist. Urgent cases were seen immediately; others were placed on waiting list.	On average, the enhanced-service group had significantly fewer days from discharge to referral and from referral to first visit than routine-service group. Enhanced-service group also received significantly more visits, significantly more minutes of therapy, and significantly more pieces of equipment. At 3 months, enhanced-service group scored significantly higher than routine-service group on Extended ADL Scale.	Possible bias from experimenter's expectations; possible selection bias (no baseline assessment of disability made); large number of dropouts in routine-service group	In short term, enhanced occupational therapy service in home may provide stroke patients with quicker improvements in functional independence and may provide health benefits to caregivers.

(continued)

Evidence Table on Occupational Therapy and Adults With Stroke: Human Studies (continued)

Author/Year	Study Objectives	Level/Design/Participants	Intervention & Outcome Measures	Results	Study Limitations	Implications for OT
			Outcomes: • Extended ADLs (Nottingham Extended ADL Scale) • ADLs (Barthel Index) • General health (General Health Questionnaire) • Equipment provided	At 6 months, enhanced-service group scored significantly higher only on mobility section of extended ADL scale. At 6 months, caregivers of enhanced-service group had significantly better general health than caregivers of routine-service group.		

Reference: Logan, P. A., Ahern, J., Gladman, J. R. F., & Lincoln, N. G. (1997). A randomized controlled trial of enhanced social service occupational therapy for stroke patients. *Clinical Rehabilitation, 11,* 107–113.

Author/Year	Study Objectives	Level/Design/Participants	Intervention & Outcome Measures	Results	Study Limitations	Implications for OT
Logan et al. (2004)	Evaluate occupational therapy intervention to improve outdoor mobility after stroke	I—Randomized controlled trial *N* = 168 (91 men, 77 women); 86 in experimental group, 82 in control group Average age: 74 years	Participants were randomly assigned to outdoor mobility intervention or control intervention. Outdoor mobility intervention involved assessment of barriers to outdoor mobility, negotiation of goals with participants, and implementation of treatment to achieve goals (providing information, recommending aids and adaptations, and building confidence). Control intervention consisted of 1 occupational therapy session focused on provision of advice, encouragement, and information. Occupational therapy intervention, delivered by occupational therapist in participants' homes, occurred in average of 4.7 visits for average total of 230 minutes.	At 4 and 10 months, experimental group members reported getting out of house as much as they would like, more than control group. They also reported undertaking significantly more journeys outdoors. At 4 months, experimental group had significantly higher mobility scores on Nottingham Extended ADL Scale than control group.	Study is of good quality.	Occupational therapy offered in stroke patients' homes and targeted at improving outdoor mobility may be effective in improving community participation.

Outcomes:
- Response to query, "Do you get out of the house as much as you would like?"
- Number of journeys outdoors in preceding month
- Extended ADLs (Nottingham Extended ADL Scale)
- Leisure activity (Nottingham Leisure Questionnaire)
- General health (short version of General Health Questionnaire)

Reference: Logan, P. A., Gladman, J. R. F., Avery, A., Walker, M. F., Dyas, J., & Groom, L. (2004). Randomised controlled trial of an occupational therapy intervention to increase outdoor mobility after stroke. *British Medical Journal, 329,* 1372–1375.

| Luke et al. (2004) | Evaluate the effectiveness of neurodevelopmental therapy to reduce upper limb impairments, activity limitations, and participation restrictions following stroke | I—Systematic review

Eight studies met the review criteria and included randomized controlled trials, single-group crossover designs, and single case design. | Neurodevelopmental treatment (Bobath concept) compared to no treatment, functional activities, Brunnstrom, wrist strengthening, motor relearning, cryotherapy, and integrated behavioral physiotherapy

Outcomes:
• Measurement of activity limitation included Barthel Index, MAS, and Action Research Arm Test
• Measures of participation included the Nottingham Health Profile
• Outcomes of impairment included shoulder pain, muscle tone, muscle strength, and motor control | At the impairment level, there was no difference between the Bobath concept and functional approach for changes in tone, muscle strength, and motor control. Those receiving the Bobath concept reported less pain than those in the cryotherapy group. Tone was reduced in the Bobath group as compared to no intervention and Brunnstrom. There were no differences between Bobath and control conditions for outcomes measuring activity limitations and participation. | Methodological quality of studies included in the review were generally poor with wide variation in number of sessions, types of clients included in studies, outcome measures used, and size of samples. | There is some evidence to support the effectiveness of Bobath interventions to reduce abnormal muscle tone after stroke but limited evidence to support its effectiveness in improving motor function, activity limitations, or participation. |

Reference: Luke, C., Dodd, K. J., & Brock, K. (2004). Outcomes of the Bobath concept on upper limb recovery following stroke. *Clinical Rehabilitation, 18,* 888–898.

(continued)

Evidence Table on Occupational Therapy and Adults With Stroke: Human Studies *(continued)*

Author/Year	Study Objectives	Level/Design/Participants	Intervention & Outcome Measures	Results	Study Limitations	Implications for OT
Ma & Trombly (2002)	Review studies of effects of occupational therapy on remediation of psychosocial, cognitive-perceptual, and sensorimotor impairments in stroke patients	I—Systematic review of 29 studies (17 randomized controlled trials, 9 nonrandomized controlled trials, 2 one-group before-and-after designs, and 1 single case study) $N = 832$ participants across 29 studies Average age: 64.3 years	Researchers reviewed studies addressing remediation of psychosocial, cognitive-perceptual, and sensorimotor impairments. Outcomes: • Depression and psychological well-being • Cognitive abilities • Learning ability • Unilateral neglect • Visual-perceptual abilities • Endurance • Range of motion and muscle strength • Organization of movement • Splinting to normalize tone or reduce spasticity	Homemaking tasks resulted in greater improvement in cognitive abilities than paper-and-pencil tasks or arts and crafts. Tasks that forced awareness of neglected space improved unilateral neglect. Coordinated movement improved when patients (1) followed written and illustrated guides for exercises, (2) used meaningful objects as targets, (3) practiced movements with specific goals, (4) moved both arms simultaneously but independently, and (5) imagined functional use of affected limb. Results for inhibitory splinting were inconclusive.	Conservative appraisal of effects because researchers excluded studies usually thought of as occupational therapy but not designated as such.	To improve cognitive abilities, therapists might use occupational tasks and activities; to improve unilateral neglect, they might cue patients to move into neglected space; to improve visual-perceptual abilities, they might require task-specific practice; to increase participation and therapeutic effect, they might use games and other meaningful activities; to increase active range of motion, patients might practice moving both arms simultaneously to accomplish specific goals; to help patients regain voluntary movement, therapists might provide written and illustrated program of exercises; to improve performance, therapists might teach patients to imagine themselves doing particular functional actions; to help patients organize movement, therapists might have them use actual objects to accomplish functional goals.

Reference: Ma, H.-I., & Trombly, C. A. (2002). A synthesis of the effects of occupational therapy for persons with stroke, part II: Remediation. *American Journal of Occupational Therapy, 56,* 260–274.

Author/Year	Study Objectives	Level/Design/Participants	Intervention & Outcome Measures	Results	Study Limitations	Implications for OT
Majid et al. (2000)	Review studies of effects of cognitive rehabilitation on memory problems in stroke patients	I—Systematic review of one randomized controlled trial $N = 12$ participants in randomized controlled study	Researchers reviewed studies of the effects of cognitive rehabilitation on memory problems in stroke patients. Their criterion for inclusion was controlled trials. Only one study met this criterion.	In the study included in the Cochrane review, cognitive rehabilitation had no significant effect on memory impairment or subjective memory complaints.	Lack of published research and small number of randomized controlled trials. Outcomes in included trial were assessed by the individual administering training.	Evidence is insufficient to support or refute effectiveness of cognitive rehabilitation for memory problems in stroke patients.

Outcomes:
- Memory function (objective measures and subjective assessment)
- Activities of daily living

Reference: Majid, M. J., Lincoln, N. B., & Weyman, N. (2000). Cognitive rehabilitation for memory deficits following stroke. *Cochrane Database of Systematic Reviews,* Issue No. 2, Art. No. CD002293.

| Mathiowetz et al. (1983) | Examine immediate effects of volar resting splint, finger spreader, firm cone, and no device on patients with hemiplegia and persons without disability | I—Counterbalanced repeated-measures design

N = 12; 4 with hemiplegia (2 men, 2 women), 8 without disability (gender not reported; control group)

Average age: Participants with hemiplegia: 43.8 years; participants without disability: not reported, range 25–40 years | Each participant squeezed a grasp meter wearing volar resting splint, finger spreader, firm cone, and no device, in succession. Once a device was put on, participant adapted for 2 minutes; squeezed for designated interval (15 seconds for participants without disability, 10 seconds for participants with hemiplegia), called grasping period; and then relaxed for 45 seconds (postgrasp period), still holding grasp meter. Device was removed, and participant rested for 2 minutes.

Participants experienced all 4 test conditions within 1 session. Occupational therapists presented conditions in laboratory.

Outcome:
• Muscle contraction as proxy for spasticity (electromyographic [EMG] measure of flexor capri radialis [FCR] and flexor digitorum profundus [FDP]) | During grasping period, for participants with hemiplegia, there were no significant differences in EMG activity among devices. However, trend of higher EMG activity was noted in both FDP and FCR for volar splint.

For participants without disability, there was significantly greater EMG activity in FCR for finger spreader compared with no device. | Possible bias from experimenters' expectations; small sample size | Occupational therapists should be cautious in providing stroke patients with positioning devices to decrease muscle spasticity, because devices may actually increase muscle activity. |

Reference: Mathiowetz, V., Bolding, D. J., & Trombly, C. A. (1983). Immediate effects of positioning devices on the normal and spastic hand measured by electromyography. *American Journal of Occupational Therapy, 37,* 247–254.

(continued)

Evidence Table on Occupational Therapy and Adults With Stroke: Human Studies (continued)

Author/Year	Study Objectives	Level/Design/Participants	Intervention & Outcome Measures	Results	Study Limitations	Implications for OT
Morris et al. (2004)	Review studies to determine effects of progressive resistance strength training (PRST) on impairment, activity limitations, and participation restrictions after stroke	I—Systematic review of 8 studies (3 randomized controlled trials, 4 before-and-after trials, and 1 single-case time-series analysis) *N* = 210 participants across 8 studies Average age: 58.3 years	Researchers reviewed trials using PRST in isolation, conducted with adult stroke patients. Outcomes: • Impairment (muscle strength, spasticity, range of movement, and depression) • Activity limitation (walking, moving from sitting to standing, stair climbing, performance of functional activities, and use of hemiparetic upper limb in functional tasks of daily living) • Social participation (roles in work, leisure, education, family, and community life) • Contextual factors (personal and environmental) and adverse events	PRST improved muscle strength. It did not seem to affect spasticity, range of movement, or depression. PRST had significant positive effects on walking. Its effects on other activities were mixed. PRST's effects on social participation were unclear. Effects of contextual factors and adverse events on outcomes were unclear.	Possible bias from exclusion of studies reported in languages other than English and studies not published or not yet completed	The results of the review provide support for PRST's efficacy in improving muscle strength and walking in adult stroke patients.

Reference: Morris, S. L., Dodd, K. J., & Morris, M. E. (2004). Outcomes of progressive resistance strength training following stroke: A systematic review. *Clinical Rehabilitation, 18,* 27–39.

Author/Year	Study Objectives	Level/Design/Participants	Intervention & Outcome Measures	Results	Study Limitations	Implications for OT
Muraki et al. (1990)	Investigate effect of sanding on cardiometabolic and pulmonary functions in patients with stroke who are elderly	II—Cohort, repeated-measures design *N* = 8 (6 men, 2 women) Average age: 67.6 years	Each participant performed exercise at five grades: grade 1—resting seated for 3 minutes on chair; grade 2—sanding horizontally (at 0 degrees) with one hand for 3 minutes with metronome at 15 cycles per minute; grade 3—doing same at 30 cycles per minute; grade 4—sanding at angle (15°) with one hand for 3 minutes at 15 cycles per minute; and grade 5—doing same at 30 cycles per minute. Participant rested for 3 minutes before starting grades 3 and 5. Participants performed under all 5 conditions in 1 session. Occupational therapist delivered intervention in hospital.	There were significant differences between grade 1 and each of the other grades, the latter producing larger values (indicating more exertion). For MET, PRP, and volume of expired air (VE), there were significant differences between grades 2 and 3. For VE, there was a significant difference between grades 4 and 5.	Possible bias from experimenters' expectations and possible maturation effect because participants were not randomly assigned to different sequences	Changing velocity of sanding may influence cardiopulmonary function more than changing angle of board. Occupational therapists might choose speed and angle according to therapeutic purpose.

Outcome:
- Cardiopulmonary function (as measured by MET level [oxygen concentration of expired air]; pressure rate product [PRP—arterial blood pressure times heart rate])

Reference: Muraki, T., Kujime, K., Su, M., Kaneko, T., & Ueba, Y. (1990). Effect of one hand sanding on cardiometabolic and ventilatory functions in the hemiplegic elderly: A preliminary investigation. *Physical and Occupational Therapy in Geriatrics, 9,* 37–48.

Study	Purpose	Design & Participants	Intervention/Outcome	Results	Limitations	Conclusions/Implications
Nelson et al. (1996)	Compare the effects of occupationally embedded exercise and rote exercise on bilaterally assisted supination	I—Randomized controlled trial N = 26 (14 men, 12 women; number per group not provided) Average age: 68.4 years	Participants were randomly assigned to occupationally embedded condition or rote condition. The occupationally embedded condition involved playing dice game that required rotation of handle. The rote condition involved same motion without dice. Participants performed 2 sets of 10 trials with 3-minute break between. Occupational therapists delivered intervention in 6 clinics. Outcome: • Supination (degree of handle rotation)	Occupationally embedded exercise resulted in significantly greater degrees of handle rotation (requiring more supination) than rote exercise.	Possible bias from experimenters' expectations	Results suggest use of occupationally embedded exercise rather than rote exercise to enhance range of motion in stroke patients.

Reference: Nelson, D. L., Konosky, K., Fleharty, K., Webb, R., Newer, K., Hazboun, V. P., et al. (1996). The effects of an occupationally embedded exercise on bilaterally assisted supination in persons with hemiplegia. *American Journal of Occupational Therapy, 50,* 639–646.

Study	Purpose	Design & Participants	Intervention/Outcome	Results	Limitations	Conclusions/Implications
Outpatient Service Trialists (2004)	Assess effects of therapy-based rehabilitation services for stroke patients who had returned home (some of whom had never been admitted to hospital)	I—Systematic review of 14 randomized trials N = 1,617 participants (gender not reported; generally balanced) across 14 trials Average age: 70 years	Researchers reviewed randomized controlled trials of outpatient services, using Cochrane Collaboration methodology. Outcomes: • Deterioration of patients' ability to undertake ADLs • Dependence in ADLs at follow-up	Therapy-based rehabilitation services significantly reduced odds of patients' deteriorating in ability to undertake ADLs and significantly improved ability to do ADLs.	Possible methodological limitations in trials reviewed; possible underestimation of effects of interventions in trials reviewed; possibility of interventions in trials reviewed not being comparable	Therapy-based rehabilitation services may be beneficial to stroke patients residing in community, though gains may be modest.

Reference: Outpatient Service Trialists. (2004). Rehabilitation therapy services for stroke patients living at home: Systematic review of randomized trials. *Lancet, 363,* 352–356.

(continued)

Evidence Table on Occupational Therapy and Adults With Stroke: Human Studies *(continued)*

Author/Year	Study Objectives	Level/Design/Participants	Intervention & Outcome Measures	Results	Study Limitations	Implications for OT
Paci (2003)	Evaluate the effectiveness of neurodevelopmental treatment for stroke survivors	I—Systematic review 15 trials were included; levels of evidence I–V with a total of 726 participants	Studies evaluating the effectiveness of studies of the Bobath concept, or neurodevelopmental treatment Outcomes: Outcome measures included MAS, functional ambulation and gait analysis, FMA scale, and Action Research Arm Test (ARAT)	While the results of review do not demonstrate the effectiveness of neurodevelopmental treatment, the methodological weaknesses of included studies limit the ability to demonstrate nonefficacy	Heterogeneity in studies with respect to age of participants and time since stroke. Many studies did not describe what was included in treatment and did not report the use of protocols for treatment. Several trials included small number of participants.	There is insufficient research evidence to support or refute the effectiveness of Bobath interventions above and beyond other treatments to improve motor function after stroke.

Reference: Paci, M. (2003). Physiotherapy based on the Bobath concept for adults with post-stroke hemiplegia: A review of effectiveness studies. *Journal of Rehabilitation Medicine, 35,* 2–7.

Author/Year	Study Objectives	Level/Design/Participants	Intervention & Outcome Measures	Results	Study Limitations	Implications for OT
Page & Levine (2006)	Determine efficacy of combining electromyography-triggered neuromuscular stimulation (ETMS) and mCIMT in treatment of patients in chronic phase of stroke	III—Before-and-after design *N* = 6 (2 men, 4 women) Average age: 62.8 years	Participants used ETMS device at home in 35-minute sessions 2 times per day 5 days per week for 8 weeks. After 1-week interval, they received mCIMT in 30-minute sessions 3 days per week for 10 weeks. They also wore slings and mitts 5 hours per day 5 days per week to restrain unaffected arm and hand. Outcomes: • Motor recovery (upper extremity motor component of FMA) • Grasp, grip, pinch, and gross movement (Action Research Arm Test) • Active wrist extension (goniometry)	Before ETMS, participants could minimally activate affected extensors but could not functionally use wrists and fingers. After ETMS, although there were no functional changes, participants had adequate active wrist extension and requisite movement in affected hand to qualify for mCIMT. After mCIMT, participants had improved ability to perform FMA wrist items and new ability to perform FMA hand items. They also had improved grasp and grip and new ability to pinch small objects.	Small sample size and lack of control group	ETMS may be useful in preparing some stroke patients for participation in CIMT.

Reference: Page, S. J., & Levine, P. (2006). Back from the brink: Electromyography-triggered stimulation combined with modified constraint-induced movement therapy in chronic stroke. *Archives of Physical Medicine and Rehabilitation, 87,* 27–31.

Study	Purpose	Design/Methods	Results	Conclusions
Page et al. (2008)	Assess the effectiveness of a reimbursable program, mCIMT on motor function in chronic stroke survivors as compared with traditional rehabilitation (proprioceptive neuromuscular facilitation; PNF) and no treatment.	I—Randomized controlled trial, comparing three groups of chronic stroke survivors: treatment group, no treatment control, and traditional rehabilitation control. N = 35 subjects, all more than 12 months poststroke, and meeting standard criteria for CIMT programs (n = 13 mCIMT, n = 12 traditional rehabilitation, n = 10 no treatment)	For a 10-week period, mCIMT participants wore a constraining mitt on the less-affected hand for 5 hours per day 5 days per week and participated in half-hour one-on-one shaping sessions 3 times per week. Traditional rehabilitation participants received the same dose of arm therapy, focusing on PNF. Control group members received no therapy. Outcomes: On completion of 10-week period • ARAT • FMA • MAL	The mCIMT group demonstrated significantly greater improvements on the MAL, FM, and ARAT as compared with the other two groups. No follow-up assessments were made to assess long-term effects. The authors speculate that the use of a behavioral contract only for the mCIMT group might have unfairly strengthened those subjects' commitment to the therapy.	This study provides additional support for mCIMT in chronic stroke survivors and, indirectly, for the efficacy of task-specific repetitive training to improve motor function in the paretic arm after stroke.

Reference: Page, S. J., Levine, P., Leonard, A., Szaflarski, J. P., & Kissela, B. M. (2008). Modified constraint-induced therapy in chronic stroke: Results of a single-blinded randomized controlled trial. *Physical Therapy, 88,* 1–8.

Study	Purpose	Design/Methods	Results	Conclusions
Pomeroy et al. (2006)	Determine the effectiveness of electrical stimulation to increase ADL function and motor ability following stroke	I—Systematic review 24 randomized controlled trials met the inclusion criteria	Trials of electrostimulation compared to no treatment, placebo, or conventional physical therapy Outcomes: • *Primary*—Functional motor ability and ADL function • *Secondary impairment*—Motor impairment and voluntary movement control	While electrostimulation resulted in some aspects of functional motor ability, motor impairment, and normality of movement as compared to no treatment, placebo, or physical therapy, the results were inconsistent. The majority of analyses contained one trial. There was variation between studies for length of time poststroke, dose of electrostimulation, and level of functional deficit. Possible selection and detection bias for the majority of trials.	There is limited evidence to support or refute the effectiveness of electrical stimulation in enhancing motor function after stroke.

Reference: Pomeroy, V. M., King, L., Pollock, A., Baily-Hallam, A., & Langhorne, P. (2006). Electrostimulation for promoting recovery of movement or functional ability after stroke. *Cochrane Database of Systematic Reviews,* Issue No. 2., Art. No. CD003241.

(continued)

Evidence Table on Occupational Therapy and Adults With Stroke: Human Studies *(continued)*

Author/Year	Study Objectives	Level/Design/Participants	Intervention & Outcome Measures	Results	Study Limitations	Implications for OT
Poole (1998)	Determine ability of stroke patients with apraxia to learn functional sequencing task (one-handed shoe tying)	II—Nonrandomized controlled trial N = 15 (gender not reported); 5 per group Average age: 71.0 years	Researcher recruited 5 stroke patients with apraxia, 5 stroke patients without apraxia from larger study, and 5 other participants (control group) from university study and family members of university faculty and students. Researcher demonstrated one-handed shoe-tying, simultaneously verbalizing instructions. Participants were assessed according to number of trials needed to tie the shoe correctly. After 5-minute interval, they were tested on retention. Intervention was delivered once by occupational therapist (author). Outcomes: • Number of trials to learn skill • Number of trials to retain skill	Control group performed significantly better on learning task than stroke patients without apraxia and stroke patients with apraxia. Stroke patients without apraxia performed significantly better on learning task than stroke patients with apraxia. Control group and stroke patients without apraxia performed significantly better on retaining task than stroke patients with apraxia. However, 4 of the 5 participants with apraxia were able to retain the task with a 5-minute delay.	Lack of randomization, small sample size, and ceiling effect on learning task (cut-off score of 5 trials)	Stroke patients with apraxia have difficulty learning and retaining functional sequencing tasks that new techniques for ADLs may require.

Reference: Poole, J. L. (1998). Effect of apraxia on the ability to learn one-handed shoe tying. *Occupational Therapy Journal of Research, 18,* 99–104.

Poole et al. (1990)	Examine effectiveness of inflatable pressure splints on motor function in stroke patients	I—Randomized controlled trial N = 18 (gender not reported); 9 per group Average age: 70.0 years	Participants were paired by scores on upper extremity section of FMA. One member of each pair was assigned to splint condition, other to nonsplint condition. Participants in both conditions received traditional occupational therapy daily. During daily sessions, participants in splint condition also wore splint 30 minutes 5 days per week for 3 weeks. Occupational therapists delivered intervention in clinics.	There were no significant differences between conditions on any measures. There was nonsignificant but moderate effect size for upper arm in nonsplint condition.	Small sample size; possible bias from experimenters' expectations of possibility of spontaneous recovery; possible unequal treatment between groups	The findings suggest that inflatable pressure splinting does not add significantly to the occupational therapy outcome of enhancing stroke patients' motor function.

Outcomes:
- Sensation
- Pain
- Motor function of upper arm, wrist, and hand (All measured by sections of FMA)

Reference: Poole, J. L., Whitney, S. L., Hangeland, N., & Baker, C. (1990). The effectiveness of inflatable pressure splints on motor function in stroke patients. *Occupational Therapy Journal of Research, 10,* 360–366.

Prange et al. (2006)	Assess the effect of robot-aided therapy on improvement of upper limb motor control and functional abilities in patients with stroke	I—Systematic review	Included interventions:	Eight studies were included in the review. The results indicated that forward-directed robot therapy improved motor control aspects such as muscle activation patterns, selectivity, and speed of movement. Long-term effect from several months to several years was demonstrated. There was no consistent impact on functional abilities.	Robotics is a promising new area of intervention to improve motor skills in chronic stroke survivors.
		The literature was searched from 1975 to 2005 in the following databases: PubMed; Cochrane Controlled Trials; Center for International Rehabilitation Research Information and Exchange; and National Rehabilitation Information Center, REHABDATA.	*Clinical trials*—Either randomized or nonrandomized controlled trials and pre- and posttests; involved stroke patients; concerned movement therapy with a robotic device	Review included studies with both subacute and chronic populations. While no qualitative differences in outcomes were noted, the number of included studies is small and makes it difficult to know if differences do exist. Except for one study controlling for time in robot-aided or conventional therapy, there was a difference in intensity between experimental and control groups.	
		Meta-analysis of pre- and posttreatment upper limb Fugl-Meyer (FM) scores for 4 studies of chronic stroke survivors also included	*Focused on upper limb motor control*—Absence of impairments in body functions (and possibly functional abilities, limitations in activities); used relevant motor control and functional ability outcome measures; published as a full-length article in a peer-reviewed journal.	The results of the meta-analysis found that robot therapy positively influenced FM scores with an average increase of 3.7 points, a 6% statistically significant increase of motor control.	
			Ten motor control and 2 functional ability measures were used in the included studies with each study measuring at least 4 different outcomes. Six studies used the upper limb portion of the FM, and 2 studies used the FIM.		

Reference: Prange, G. B., Jannink, M.J.A, Groothuis-Oudshoorn, C.G.M., Hermens, H. J., & IJzerman, M. J. (2006). Systematic review of the effect of robot-aided therapy on recovery of the hemiparetic arm after stroke. *Journal of Rehabilitation Research and Development, 43,* 171–184.

(continued)

Evidence Table on Occupational Therapy and Adults With Stroke: Human Studies (continued)

Author/Year	Study Objectives	Level/Design/Participants	Intervention & Outcome Measures	Results	Study Limitations	Implications for OT
Price & Pandyan (2000)	Evaluate the efficacy of electrical stimulation to prevent or treat shoulder pain following stroke	I—Systematic review 4 randomized controlled trials met the inclusion criteria	All randomized controlled trials that assessed electrical stimulation, including functional electrical stimulation and transcutaneous electrical nerve stimulation applied any time following stroke. Outcomes: • Presence of pain • Intensity of pain	The results of the studies indicate that there was no significant change in pain incidence or intensity, upper limb motor recovery, or upper limb spasticity. There was, however, a significant improvement in pain-free range of passive humeral lateral rotation following electrical stimulation that may be due to a reduction in severity of glenohumeral subluxation.	Numbers in individual studies included in the review were small. Quality of some studies included in the review was less than optimal.	Electrical stimulation may be effective in improving shoulder subluxation and pain-free passive range of motion in lateral rotation.

Reference: Price, C. I. M., & Pandyan, A. D. (2000). Electrical stimulation for preventing and treating poststroke shoulder pain. *Cochrane Database of Systematic Reviews,* Issue No 4., Art. No. CD001698.

Author/Year	Study Objectives	Level/Design/Participants	Intervention & Outcome Measures	Results	Study Limitations	Implications for OT
Ro et al. (2006)	Determine feasibility of using TMS to assess functional motor reorganization after CIMT in patients in subacute phase of stroke; determine feasibility, safety, and effectiveness of using constraint-induced movement therapy with patients in subacute phase of stroke; and determine whether brain reorganization of movement control correlates with improved motor function	I—Randomized controlled trial *N* = 8 participants (5 men, 3 women), all within 2 weeks after stroke; 4 in group receiving constraint-induced movement therapy and 4 in control group Average age: 61.4 years	Participants were randomly assigned to group receiving CIMT or control group. CIMT includes contraint to unaffected hand (by wearing a mitt) during 90% of waking hours and intensive task-based practice sessions using shaping. Control group received traditional therapy, focused on increasing function with use of both hands. Therapy, delivered by 1 occupational therapist and 1 physical therapist in laboratory, occurred 3 hours per day 6 days per week for 14 consecutive days.	At 3-month follow-up, constraint-induced movement therapy group showed significantly larger representations for movement than control group showed. At end of treatment and 3-month follow-up, constraint-induced movement therapy group was significantly faster in motor performance on Grooved Pegboard Test (GPT) than control group and scored significantly higher on FMA.	Small sample size	TMS can safely and effectively assess brain function in patients in subacute state of stroke. CIMT may enhance motor reorganization and accelerate motor recovery when started within 2 weeks following stroke.

Outcomes:
- Location and extent of motor representation of hand movement (TMS)
- Motor performance (GPT; FMA)
- Amount of use and quality of movement (MAL)

At 3-month follow-up, performance on GPT and FMA was significantly and highly correlated with motor representation of impaired hand.

There were no differences in performance on the MAL between groups at any stage of the study.

Reference: Ro, T., Noser, E., Boake, C., Johnson, R., Gaber, M., Speroni, A., et al. (2006). Functional reorganization and recovery after constraint-induced movement therapy in subacute stroke: Case reports. Neurocase, 12, 50–60.

| Roth et al. (1998) | Study association between neurological functioning and ability to perform ADLs in stroke patients and study degree of disability reduction in patients who do not have reduction in impairment levels | I—Prospective cohort design N = 402 (183 men, 219 women) Average age: 64.5 years | Researchers compared participants' scores on admission to and discharge from rehabilitation hospital. Average length of stay was 30.5 days. Outcomes: • Impairment (National Institutes of Health Stroke Scale [NIHSS]) • Motor and cognitive disability (FIM) | Participants made significant gains in motor and cognitive ability between admission and discharge. Gains in motor ability were significantly greater than gains in cognitive ability. There were significant (but small) correlations between impairment and disability. Relationships with motor disability were stronger than those with cognitive disability. Patients who did not experience reduction in impairment levels showed significant (but small) decrease in disability, as did patients who did experience reduction in impairment levels. | Possible lack of sensitivity in NIHSS to small changes in improvement and failure of NIHSS to measure some clinically important changes. Impairment and disability are correlated, but rehabilitation can improve disability (performance of self-care tasks) even when impairments cannot be improved. |

Reference: Roth, E. J., Heinemann, A. W., Lovell, L. L., Harvey, R. L., McGuire, J. R., & Diaz, S. (1998). Impairment and disability: Their relation during stroke rehabilitation. Archives of Physical Medicine and Rehabilitation, 79, 329–335.

(continued)

Evidence Table on Occupational Therapy and Adults With Stroke: Human Studies (continued)

Author/Year	Study Objectives	Level/Design/Participants	Intervention & Outcome Measures	Results	Study Limitations	Implications for OT
Smedley et al. (1986)	Compare effectiveness of novel, entertaining exercise and traditional therapy with stroke patients	II—Nonrandomized controlled trial $N = 50$ participants (gender not reported); 25 per group Average age: Not reported; range 40–84 years	Stroke inpatients at one hospital were designated as experimental group, stroke inpatients at another hospital as control group. Both groups received traditional occupational therapy. Experimental group also used slot machines adapted to operate with slugs and to allow graded resistive exercises. Occupational therapists delivered interventions in 2 hospitals. Outcomes: • Range of motion • Muscle strength • Gross motor coordination • Fine motor coordination • Depression (Beck Depression Inventory)	Experimental group improved significantly more than control group on all measures.	Possibility that findings are not conclusive because study used research design where the 2 groups were at different hospitals, and therapists may have known research hypothesis; possible selection bias (chronicity, site of lesion); unequal treatments.	Incorporating an entertaining and novel treatment may be more effective than traditional intervention.

Reference: Smedley, R. R., Fiorino, A. J., Soucar, E., Reynolds, D., Smedley, W. P., & Aronica, M. J. (1986). Slot machines: Their use in rehabilitation after stroke. *Archives of Physical Medicine and Rehabilitation, 67*, 546–549.

Author/Year	Study Objectives	Level/Design/Participants	Intervention & Outcome Measures	Results	Study Limitations	Implications for OT
Söderback (1988)	Evaluate effectiveness and maintenance of occupational therapy training of intellectual functions	I—Randomized controlled trial $N = 67$ (35 men, 32 women); 15 in intellectual function training (IFT) plus regular rehabilitation (RR) group, 19 in intellectual housework training (IHT) plus RR group, 15 in IFT plus IHT plus RR group, and 18 in RR group (control) Average age: 47.0 years	Participants were randomly assigned to group receiving IFT (paper-and-pencil cognitive exercises) plus RR (crafts, hobbies, and newspaper reading); group receiving IHT (homemaking activities to improve cognition) plus RR; group receiving IFT plus IHT plus RR; or group receiving RR only (control group). IFT plus RR received average of 37 1-hour sessions; IHT plus RR received average of 16 2.5-hour sessions; IFT plus IHT plus RR received average of 22 sessions (14 1-hour sessions of IFT and 8 2.5-hour sessions of IHT); and RR received average of 43 hours over 79 days.	There were significant differences between groups with IHA: • Between IFT plus RR, and RR: attention subtest • Between IHT plus RR, and RR: verbal and memory subtests • Between IFT plus IHT plus RR, and RR: verbal, memory, and logical subtests There were no significant differences among three experimental groups and RR on IFA.	Possibility of spontaneous recovery; possible equivalence of treatment (IFT and RR); use of multiple statistical tests without correction	Both paper-and-pencil tasks and functional tasks encountered in daily life may be effective in improving cognitive function in stroke survivors.

Occupational therapists delivered interventions in clinics.

Outcome:
• Various components of cognition—for example, verbal understanding, verbal fluency, ability to process and organize visual input, ability to relate items in space, attention, problem solving, and ability to work with numbers (Intellectual Function Assessment [IFA], Intellectual Housework Assessment [IHA])

Reference: Söderback, I. (1988). The effectiveness of training intellectual functions in adults with acquired brain damage: An evaluation of occupational therapy methods. *Scandinavian Journal of Rehabilitation Medicine, 20,* 47–56.

| Sterr et al. (2002) | Compare the effectiveness of 3-hour versus 6-hour daily training sessions in CIMT | I—Randomized controlled trial, comparing 2 groups of CIMT participants. Fifteen adults with chronic hemiparesis (13 poststroke; n = 8 [3-hour group], n = 7 [6-hour group]). Repeated measures were administered on 2 occasions before treatment, immediately following the standard 2-week CIMT intervention, and on 2 occasions weekly following CIMT. | Participants in a CIMT program were randomly assigned to shaping sessions whose duration was either 3 hours per day or 6 hours per day (6 hours is standard in CIMT protocols). Outcomes: • MAL • WMFT | MAL scores improved significantly posttreatment for both groups and remained well above baseline level during follow-up. WMFT scores improved significantly, using a two-tailed test, for the group receiving 6-hour daily shaping sessions. For the group receiving 3-hour daily shaping sessions, WMFT scores improved significantly, using a one-tailed test. | Small sample size | Shaping sessions of 3 hours per day in a CIMT protocol may be effective in improving motor function in patients with chronic hemiparesis, but the standard protocol of 6 hours per day of directed task practice is more effective in improving motor function. |

Reference: Sterr, A., Elbert, T., Berthold, I., Kolbel, S., Rockstroh, B., & Taub, E. (2002). Longer versus shorter daily constraint-induced movement therapy of chronic hemiparesis: An exploratory study. *Archives of Physical Medicine and Rehabilitation, 83,* 1374–1377.

| Steultjens et al. (2003) | Review studies of effects of occupational therapy with stroke patients | I—Systematic review of 32 studies (18 randomized controlled trials, 6 case-control trials, and 8 controlled designs) | Researchers reviewed literature on effectiveness of occupational therapy with stroke patients. They then conducted meta-analyses or synthesized best evidence by intervention category: comprehensive occupational therapy, training of sensorimotor functions, training of cognitive functions, training of skills (dressing, cooking, | *Comprehensive occupational therapy:* High-quality studies showed small but significant effects on primary ADLs, extended ADLs, and social participation. *Training of sensorimotor functions:* High-quality studies showed no significant effects on primary ADLs, extended | Variability in interventions across settings and countries | Comprehensive occupational therapy is effective in improving primary ADLs, extended ADLs, and social participation. Skill training may be effective in improving primary ADLs. Training in cognitive functions may improve visual perception. Evidence is insufficient to support splinting to decrease muscle tone. |

(continued)

Evidence Table on Occupational Therapy and Adults With Stroke: Human Studies *(continued)*

Author/Year	Study Objectives	Level/Design/Participants	Intervention & Outcome Measures	Results	Study Limitations	Implications for OT
			etc.), advice and instruction regarding assistive devices, provision of splints, and education of family or primary caregiver. Outcomes: • Primary ADLs • Extended ADLs • Social participation • Arm and hand function • Muscle tone • Cognitive functions	ADLs, social participation, or arm and hand function. Training of cognitive functions: One low-quality randomized controlled trial suggested that visual scanning and visual-spatial ability improve. Training of skills: One high-quality study showed significant improvement in primary ADLs. Advice and instruction regarding assistive devices: One high-quality study showed no significant results. Provision of splints: Five low-quality studies showed no significant results. Education of family or primary caregiver: No occupational therapy studies focused on this intervention.		

Reference: Steultjens, E. M. J., Dekker, J., Bouter, L. M., van de Nes, J. C. M., Cup, E. H. D., & van den Ende, C. H. M. (2003). Occupational therapy for stroke patients: A systematic review. *Stroke, 34,* 676–687.

Author/Year	Study Objectives	Level/Design/Participants	Intervention & Outcome Measures	Results	Study Limitations	Implications for OT
Szaflarski et al. (2006)	Determine whether cortical changes occur in patients in chronic phase of stroke following mCIMT	III—Before-and-after design *N* = 14 (7 men, 7 women); 4 with stroke, 10 without disability Average age: 59.3 years	Stroke patients received mCIMT 30 minutes per day 3 times per week for 10 weeks. Therapy was delivered by an occupational therapist. Patients wore mitt on unaffected hand 5 hours per day for same 10 weeks. Participants without disability acted as control group for data on typical activation patterns in finger-tapping tasks.	Three of 4 stroke patients showed cortical reorganization on *f* MRI. Same 3 showed increases in motor function, reductions in impairment, and increases in amount and quality of use.	Small sample size, lack of randomization, and lack of true control group	mCIMT appears to induce cortical reorganization. In patients who responded to therapy, cortical reorganization was positively related to degree of increase in use of affected arm and in ability.

Outcomes:
- Cortical reorganization (fMRI)
- Motor function (FMA)
- Impairment (ARAT)
- Amount and quality of use (MAL)

Reference: Szaflarski, J. P., Page, S. P., Kissela, B. M., Lee, J.-H., Levine, P., & Strakowski, S. M. (2006). Cortical reorganization following modified constraint-induced movement therapy: A study of 4 patients with chronic stroke. *Archives of Physical Medicine and Rehabilitation, 87,* 1052–1058.

| Taub et al. (2006) | Conduct placebo-controlled trial of CIMT with patients in chronic phase of stroke | II—Nonrandomized controlled trial

$N = 41$ (27 men, 14 women); 21 in CIMT group, 20 in control group

Average age: 52.7 years | Participants were assigned in blocks to CIMT group or control group, on basis of scores on WMFT (to match groups on initial motor deficit). CIMT includes constraint to unaffected hand (by wearing a mitt) during 90% of waking hours and intensive task based practice sessions using shaping. Control group participated in fitness program (exercises and games). Treatment occurred 6 hours per day, 5 days per week, for 2 weeks.

Outcomes:
- Quality of movement (QOM scale of MAL)
- Actual amount of use (upper-extremity actual-amount-of-use test)
- Motor ability (speed and quality; performance-time and functional-ability scales of WMFT) | CIMT group showed significantly greater improvement in quality of movement (on MAL), actual amount of use, and speed.

At 4-week follow-up, CIMT group had retained gains on MAL.

At 2-year follow-up, constraint-induced movement therapy group showed only 23% decrease from MAL levels immediately following treatment. | Lack of randomization | CIMT is effective in rehabilitating upper-extremity motor function in chronic stroke survivors. |

Reference: Taub, E., Uswatte, G., King, D. K., Morris, D., Crago, J. E., & Chatterjee, A. (2006). A placebo-controlled trial of constraint-induced movement therapy for upper extremity after stroke. *Stroke, 37,* 1045–1049.

(continued)

Author/Year	Study Objectives	Level/Design/Participants	Intervention & Outcome Measures	Results	Study Limitations	Implications for OT
Tham & Tegnér (1997)	Compare effects of video feedback and conventional verbal feedback on patients' unilateral-neglect behavior when performing practical tasks and assess extent to which any observed effect generalizes to other tasks	II—Nonrandomized controlled trial $N = 14$ (11 men, 3 women); 7 per group Average age: 67.9 years	Researchers recruited consecutive series of 14 patients and assigned first 7 to video feedback and second 7 to conventional verbal feedback. Both groups were tested once on day 1 and twice on day 2, each time with 4 tests for unilateral neglect (see below). On day 2, after first test on Baking Tray Task, video-feedback group received video feedback on performance, and conventional-feedback group received verbal feedback. Then, with both groups, therapist discussed compensatory strategies and offered instruction in use of tactile discrimination to locate left edge of tray. Three hours later, both groups were tested again. Outcomes: • Symmetrical placement of "buns" (wood blocks) on tray (Baking Tray Task) • Marking of 40 lines of equal length in random display (Line Cancellation Task) • Copying of figure (Figure Copying Task) • Bisection of 15 lines of 3 lengths presented in random order	Video-feedback group improved significantly on Baking Tray Task after feedback. Neither group showed generalization from training on Baking Tray Task to performance on other tests.	Lack of randomization; possible selection bias (video feedback group included no women; conventional feedback group included 3 women)	Video feedback may be useful in rehabilitating patients with unilateral neglect.

Reference: Tham, K., & Tegnér, R. (1997). Video feedback in the rehabilitation of patients with unilateral neglect. *Archives of Physical Medicine and Rehabilitation, 78,* 410–413.

Thielman et al. (2004)	Evaluate effects of 2 rehabilitative approaches on reaching in stroke patients	I—Randomized controlled trial $N = 12$ (5 men, 7 women); 6 per group Average age: 72.8 years	Participants were matched on Motor Assessment Scale (MAS) scores; one of each pair was randomly assigned to task-related training (TRT), the other to progressive resistive exercise (PRE). Participants were categorized as being at high or low functional level. TRT involved training to touch or grasp various objects on different surfaces. PRE involved pulling with whole arm against resistive tubing. Interventions, delivered by physical therapist in participants' homes, occurred in 35-minute sessions 12 times across 4 weeks. Outcomes: • Trunk use (compensatory strategy; Peak Performance System) • Arm trajectories (Peak Performance System) • Function level (MAS and arm section of Rivermead Stroke Assessment)	Low-level TRT participants significantly increased trunk use to touch ipsilateral objects; low-level PRE participants significantly increased trunk use to touch midline and contralateral objects. Low-level TRT participants significantly straightened hand paths and significantly improved on RSA. Low-level PRE participants did neither. High-level TRT participants showed no change in trunk use, whereas high-level PRE participants significantly decreased trunk use to touch ipsilateral objects.	Study is of good quality. Training benefits may depend on initial level of functioning. Low-level patients may benefit more from TRT, while high-level patients may benefit more from PRE.

Reference: Thielman, G. T., Dean, C. M., & Gentile, A. M. (2004). Rehabilitation of reaching after stroke: Task-related training versus progressive resistive exercise. *Archives of Physical Medicine and Rehabilitation, 85,* 1613–1618.

Trombly & Ma (2002)	Review studies of effects of occupational therapy on restoration of role, task, and activity performance in stroke patients	I—Systematic review of 15 studies (10 randomized controlled trials, 2 nonrandomized controlled trials, and 3 one-group before-and-after designs) $N = 895$ participants across 15 studies Average age: 70.3 years	Researchers reviewed studies addressing restoration of roles, tasks, or activities. Outcomes: • Participation in life roles • Activity—instrumental or extended ADLs • Activity—basic ADLs	Role participation, ADLs, and IADLs improved significantly more for intervention conditions than for control conditions. Effect of role participation appeared to depend on dosage and goal specificity. More frequent treatment and more specific goals produced significant positive effects. Task-specific training in instrumental or extended ADLs in home appeared to	Conservative appraisal of effects because researchers usually excluded studies thought of as occupational therapy but not designated as such To improve stroke patients' performance, therapists might use structured instruction in specific, client-identified activities, appropriate adaptations, practice within familiar context, and feedback.

(continued)

Evidence Table on Occupational Therapy and Adults With Stroke: Human Studies *(continued)*

Author/Year	Study Objectives	Level/Design/Participants	Intervention & Outcome Measures	Results	Study Limitations	Implications for OT
				result in improved ADL performance.		
				Task-specific practice of basic ADLs that patients identified as important appeared to result in improved performance.		

Reference: Trombly, C. A., & Ma, H.-I. (2002). A synthesis of the effects of occupational therapy on persons with stroke, part I: Restoration of roles, tasks, and activities. *American Journal of Occupational Therapy, 56,* 250–259.

Author/Year	Study Objectives	Level/Design/Participants	Intervention & Outcome Measures	Results	Study Limitations	Implications for OT
Trombly & Quintana (1983)	Examine effect of five types of exercise on finger extension of stroke patients	I—Randomized controlled trial; repeated-measures design *N* = 10 (gender not reported) Average age: 53.1 years	Participants were randomly assigned to 1 of 4 groups, each group representing different sequence of 5 exercises: resisted grasp, resisted extension, unresisted grasp and release, unresisted rapid extension, and unresisted slow extension. Participants performed 3 repetitions of each exercise with 2-minute rest in between exercises, all within 1 day. Occupational therapists delivered intervention in laboratory. Outcomes: • Activity of extensor digitorum (ED), flexor digitorum superficialis (FDS), and flexor digitorum profundus (FDP) (measured electronically) • Total range of motion of finger extension, adding together degrees of movement of metacarpophalangeal and proximal interphalangeal joints of middle finger during opening from full flexion	During resisted extension, participants used ED at significantly higher percentage than they used FDP, but not at significantly higher percentage than they used FDS. During rapid extension, participants used ED at significantly higher percentage than they used FDS, but not at significantly higher percentage than they used FDP. During slow extension, participants used ED at significantly higher percentage than they used either FDS or FDP. During resisted grasp, participants used all three muscles at high percentage, none significantly higher than others. During unresisted grasp, participants used no muscle at significantly higher percentage than others. During release, however, they used ED at significantly higher percentage than they used either FDS or FDP.	Possible bias from experimenters' expectations	Occupational therapists might use exercise to facilitate hand muscle activity in stroke patients. They should choose type of exercise according to therapeutic purpose.

118

Adults With Stroke

| | | | | | Participants showed no significant changes in range of motion of finger extension. |

Reference: Trombly, C. A., & Quintana, L. A. (1983). The effects of exercise on finger extension of CVA patients. *American Journal of Occupational Therapy, 37,* 195–202.

| Trombly et al. (1986) | Examine effects of three exercises on finger extension | I—Randomized controlled trial

N = 20 (9 men, 11 women); 5 per group

Average age: 66.8 years | Study involved 4 conditions: ballistic extension, resisted extension, resisted grasp, and control. Participants were randomly assigned to conditions; 2 patients who could grasp but not actively release were assigned to grasp task.

In first 3 conditions, participants performed exercise 10 times per session for 1 session per day for 20 treatment days. Occupational therapists delivered treatments in clinic.

Outcomes:
• Active range of motion of finger extension
• Tapping (involving ability to reverse movement rapidly, proxy measure for spasticity)
• Grasp/release | Ballistic- and resisted-extension groups improved significantly more than resisted- grasp and control groups in ability to reverse movement rapidly (indicating decreased spasticity).

Groups showed no significant differences in abilities to grasp and release or in active finger extension. | Imbalance in participant assignment, resulting in significantly more patients in ballistic- and resisted-extension groups at higher level of recovery of motor control; possible bias from experimenters' expectations | Occupational therapists might use extension exercises to improve finger extensions of stroke patients. They also might incorporate such exercises in home programs. |

Reference: Trombly, C. A., Thayer-Nason, L., Bliss, G., Girard, C. A., Lyrist, L. A., & Brexa-Hooson, A. (1986). The effectiveness of therapy in improving finger extension in stroke patients. *American Journal of Occupational Therapy, 40,* 612–617.

| Trombly & Wu (1999) | Examine effects of task demands and contextual constraints on movement in stroke patients | I—Randomized controlled trial; counterbalanced repeated-measures design

N = 14 (9 men, 5 women)

Average age: 65.0 years | Experiment 1: Participants were randomly assigned to AB or BA sequence of conditions. Condition A involved reaching for preferred food on plate on table at midline; condition B, reaching forward to center of empty plate.

Experiment 2: Participants were randomly assigned to ABC, BCA, CAB, ACB, BAC, or CBA sequence of conditions. Condition A, natural context, involved reaching for the | Experiment 1: Participants showed significantly smoother, faster, more preplanned, and more forceful movements under condition A than under condition B.

Experiment 2: Participants showed no significant differences among conditions. | Study is of good quality. | Findings support occupational therapy practice of using objects in functional context to improve coordinated movement. |

(continued)

Evidence Table on Occupational Therapy and Adults With Stroke: Human Studies *(continued)*

Author/Year	Study Objectives	Level/Design/Participants	Intervention & Outcome Measures	Results	Study Limitations	Implications for OT
			receiver on an active telephone and dialing a number. Condition B, partial context, involved reaching for a receiver only (detached from telephone cord and base). Condition C, simulated condition, involved reaching for a wooden stick of the same size, weight, and color as receiver. Participants performed 10 trials per condition for 2 experiments within 1 day. Conditions were presented by experimenter in laboratory. Outcomes: • Smoothness (number of crossings of zero line in acceleration profile) • Speed (movement time) • Directness (displacement from straight line) • Force (peak velocity) • Planning strategy (location of peak velocity in velocity profile)			

Reference: Trombly, C. A., & Wu, C.-Y. (1999). Effect of rehabilitation tasks on organization of movement after stroke. *American Journal of Occupational Therapy, 53,* 333–344.

Author/Year	Study Objectives	Level/Design/Participants	Intervention & Outcome Measures	Results	Study Limitations	Implications for OT
Turton & Fraser (1990)	Examine effectiveness of home therapy programs in improving reaching movement in stroke patients	II—Nonrandomized controlled trial N = 22 (12 men, 10 women); 12 in experimental group, 10 in control group Average age: 58.0 years	Participants were assigned to home therapy group or control group in alternate runs of 5. The home therapy group received a booklet and written and illustrated program of exercises considered appropriate to participants' individual stages of recovery. Participants performed exercises 2–3 times per day for an average of 9 weeks. Therapist visited occasionally to adjust program.	Experimental group showed significantly more improvement on peg test than control group. There were no significant differences between groups on motor assessment.	Possibility of cointervention (some patients also receiving outpatient therapy) confounding results; possible bias from therapist's expectations; ceiling effects on motor assessment (some patients scored maximum on pretest and thus not able to improve); and floor effects on peg test (some patients did not have sufficient motor activity to attempt test).	Although the findings are inconclusive due to study limitations, incorporating home exercise programs into the treatment of stroke patients may be important. Programs should be appropriate to each patient's stage each of recovery and individual problems.

Control group received no treatment. Therapist visited control group at home for assessment only.

Outcome:
- Sensorimotor performance (upper-limb activity assessment of Southern Motor Group's motor assessment and Ten-Hole Peg Test)

Reference: Turton, A., & Fraser, C. (1990). The use of home therapy programmes for improving recovery of the upper limb following stroke. *British Journal of Occupational Therapy, 53,* 457–462.

| Underwood et al. (2006) | Explore relationship between intensity of CIMT and fatigue and pain | I—Randomized controlled trial

$N = 32$ (22 men, 10 women); 18 in subacute group, 14 in chronic group

Average age: 61.6 years | Participants were randomly assigned to a group that would receive therapy during subacute phase of stroke or a group that would receive therapy during chronic phase of stroke, using a process designed to ensure balance between groups in functional capability, sex, hemiplegic side, and hand dominance. The subacute group received CIMT 3–9 months after stroke; the chronic therapy group received therapy 1 year after enrollment in study. Both groups received therapy 6 hours per day for 10 days. Therapy relied on shaping and repetitive practice.

Outcomes:
• Upper extremity motor function (WMFT)
• Upper extremity joint pain (FMA)
• Intensity of therapy (minutes actually spent in task practice)
• Fatigue and pain during training (single-item rating scales of 1–10) | Both groups showed significant improvement in motor function from before therapy to after therapy.

Both groups achieved same intensity of therapy.

For both groups, there was no change in morning or afternoon pain and fatigue during treatment period. | Small sample size | CIMT can improve motor function in patients in subacute or chronic phase of stroke with minimal to moderate impairment. With careful screening, neither pain nor fatigue should be of concern in using CIMT with these patients. |

Reference: Underwood, J., Clark, P. C., Blanton, S., Aycock, D. M., & Wolf, S. L. (2006). Pain, fatigue, and intensity of practice in people with stroke who are receiving constraint-induced movement therapy. *Physical Therapy, 86,* 1241–1250.

(continued)

Evidence Table on Occupational Therapy and Adults With Stroke: Human Studies *(continued)*

Author/Year	Study Objectives	Level/Design/Participants	Intervention & Outcome Measures	Results	Study Limitations	Implications for OT
Uswatte et al. (2006)	Evaluate effect of type of training provided to affected arm and type of restraint used on unaffected arm in CIMT with patients in chronic phase of stroke	II—Nonrandomized control trial *N* = 17 (10 men, 7 women); 4 in sling-and-task-practice group, 4 in sling-and-shaping group, 5 in half-glove-and-shaping group, and 4 in shaping-only group Average age: 63.8 years	Participants were consecutively assigned to sling-and-task-practice group, sling-and-shaping group, half-glove-and-shaping group, and shaping-only group. Sling-and-task-practice group engaged in repetitive practice of functional tasks (eating lunch, throwing ball, etc.). 6 hours per day for 10 consecutive weekdays. Sling-and-shaping group received shaping of affected-arm use on same schedule. In both groups, movement of unaffected arm was restricted by splint/sling combination for target of 90% of waking hours. Half-glove-and-shaping group received same treatment as sling-and-shaping group but wore half-glove rather than splint/sling combination. Shaping-only group received shaping of affected arm on same schedule as other groups but wore no restraint. Therapy was delivered in laboratory by therapists (type not reported). Outcomes: • Real-world arm use (Quality of Movement Scale of MAL) • Motor ability (WMFT)	Immediately following treatment, all 4 groups combined showed significant improvement in real-world arm use from before treatment to after treatment. All 4 combined also showed significant improvement in motor ability. Further, there were no significant differences among groups. One month after treatment, all 4 groups combined continued to show significant gains in real-world arm use from before treatment to after treatment. There were no significant differences among groups. Two years after treatment, 3 groups combined (shaping-only excluded because of missing data) still showed significant gains in real-world arm use from before treatment to after treatment.	Possible bias from difference in training intensity; possible confounding from similarity of task practice to shaping; possible confounding from failure to monitor compliance with wearing of restraint; small sample size; lack of no-treatment group	In terms of immediate outcomes, shaping and task practice may be equivalent methods for training affected arm. Physical restraint of unaffected arm may not be necessary to promote use of affected arm. Other components of therapy (training of affected arm, contract with patient, etc.) may suffice.

Reference: Uswatte, G., Taub, E., Morris, D., Barman, J., & Crago, J. (2006). Contribution of the shaping and restraint components of constraint-induced movement therapy to treatment outcome. *NeuroRehabilitation, 21,* 147–156.

Study	Purpose	Design / Participants	Methods / Outcomes	Results	Limitations	Conclusions
van Heugten et al. (1998)	Evaluate outcome of therapy program for stroke patients with apraxia	III—Before-and-after design N = 33 (18 men, 15 women) Average age: 70.1 years	Researchers recruited stroke patients with apraxia from general hospitals, rehabilitation centers, and nursing homes. Participants learned strategies to compensate for apraxia. Participants were assessed before and after treatment. Treatment, delivered by occupational therapists in facilities from which participants were recruited, occurred for 12 weeks. Therapists determined number of sessions per week (length of sessions not indicated). Outcomes: • Motor functioning (short test consisting of 8 tasks) • Apraxia (test of apraxia based on tests of De Renzi) • ADL (standardized observations, Barthel Index, ADL questionnaire)	Participants improved significantly in motor functioning, apraxia, and ADLs. Effect size for ADLs was large compared with effect sizes for apraxia and motor functioning.	Lack of randomization; no control group; and variation across participants in number of treatments received per week	Therapy focused on strategies to compensate for apraxia, rather than on recovery from apraxia, may help stroke patients function more independently.

Reference: van Heugten, C. M., Dekker, J., Deelman, J., Deelman, B. G., van Dijk, A. J., Stehmann-Saris, J. C., & Kinebanian, A. (1998). Outcome of strategy training in stroke patients with apraxia: A phase II study. *Clinical Rehabilitation, 12*, 294–303.

Study	Purpose	Design / Participants	Methods / Outcomes	Results	Limitations	Conclusions
van Heugten et al. (2000)	Investigate which additional cognitive and motor impairments were present in stroke patients with apraxia and which of them influenced effects of treatment	II—Nonrandomized controlled trial N = 69 (32 men, 37 women); 33 in experimental group, 36 in control group Average age: 64.8 years	Researchers recruited stroke patients with apraxia (experimental group) and stroke patients without apraxia (control group) from 3 general hospitals, 8 rehabilitation centers, and 5 nursing homes. Experimental group received treatment in use of compensatory strategies. Treatment, delivered by occupational therapists in facilities from which participants were recruited, occurred in 2–5 sessions per week (length of sessions not indicated) for 12 weeks.	Before treatment, the experimental group scored significantly lower than control group on apraxia, language comprehension, cognitive orientation, and short-term memory. Both groups scored poorly on motor functioning. Following treatment, the experimental group improved significantly on apraxia, motor functioning, and ADLs. Effect size for ADLs was large compared with effect sizes for apraxia and motor functioning.	Lack of randomization and possible selection bias (from experimental group being significantly younger than control group)	Apraxia is associated with additional cognitive and motor impairments. Therapy focused on strategies to compensate for apraxia, rather than on recovery from apraxia, may help stroke patients function more independently. Effect of training may be stronger in more severely disabled patients.

(continued)

Evidence Table on Occupational Therapy and Adults With Stroke: Human Studies (*continued*)

Author/Year	Study Objectives	Level/Design/Participants	Intervention & Outcome Measures	Results	Study Limitations	Implications for OT
			Control group received no intervention. Outcomes: • Apraxia (test of apraxia based on tests of De Renzi) • Motor functioning (short test based on other tests, such as motricity index) • ADLs (4 standardized observations) • Language comprehension (Comprehension of Sentences subtest of SAN-test) • Cognitive orientation (Cognitive Screening Test) • Unilateral visual neglect (Star Cancellation subtest of Behavioural Inattention Test) • Short-term memory (digit-span test)	On apraxia and ADL observations, participants who were more severely impaired showed most marked improvement in independent functioning.		

Reference: van Heugten, C. M., Dekker, J., Deelman, B. G., Stehmann-Saris, J. C., & Kinebanian, A. (2000). Rehabilitation of stroke patients with apraxia: The role of additional cognitive and motor impairments. *Disability and Rehabilitation, 22,* 547–554.

Author/Year	Study Objectives	Level/Design/Participants	Intervention & Outcome Measures	Results	Study Limitations	Implications for OT
Van Peppen et al. (2004)	Review studies of effects of physical therapy on functional outcomes in stroke patients	I—Systematic review of 151 studies (123 randomized controlled trials and 28 controlled clinical trials) *N* = 9,139 participants across 151 studies	Researchers reviewed studies of effects of physical therapy on functional outcomes in stroke patients. They then analyzed studies by intervention category: traditional neurological treatment approaches; training of sensorimotor function or influencing of muscle tone; training for cardiovascular fitness and aerobic capacity; training for mobility and mobility-related activities; exercises for upper limb; biofeedback; functional electrical stimulation (FES) and neuromuscular stimulation (NMS); provision of orthotics and assistive devices; treatment	Intense exercise training, aerobic training, transcutaneous electrical nerve stimulation, constraint-induced movement therapy, training for sit-to-stand transfers, NMS for glenohumeral subluxation, external auditory rhythms during gait training, and treadmill training produced significant effects. Impairment-focused programs produced significant improvements in range of motion, muscle power, and reduction of muscle tone but failed to generalize to activities.	Methodological flaws in most studies reviewed and small number of participants in most studies reviewed	Findings support the use of interventions to improve performance as well as capacity to perform ADLs after stroke, particularly when intervention is intensive and begins soon after onset.

			of shoulder pain and hand edema; and provision of more intense exercise therapy.		Insufficient or no evidence was found for traditional neurological treatment approaches, exercises for upper limb, biofeedback, FES or NMS to improve dexterity or gait, provision of orthotics and assistive devices, or interventions to reduce shoulder pain and hand edema.

Reference: Van Peppen, R. P. Kwakkel, G., Wood-Dauphinee, S., Hendriks, H. J., Van der Wees, P. J., & Dekker, J. (2004). The impact of physical therapy on functional outcomes after stroke: What's the evidence? *Clinical Rehabilitation, 18,* 833–862.

| Walker et al. (1996) | Examine effectiveness of dressing practice for stroke patients after discharge from hospital | I—Randomized controlled trial; crossover design

N = 30 (16 men, 14 women); 15 per group

Average age: 68.0 years | Participants were randomly assigned to receive no interventions for 3 months and then treatment for 3 months, or vice versa. Treatment involved instructing participants and caregivers in appropriate techniques, such as dressing affected limb first, conserving energy, and using red thread to mark alignment of buttons, and advising participants and caregivers on choice of clothing.

Intervention, delivered by occupational therapist in participants' homes, occurred for 3 months; study lasted 6 months. Amount of therapy was at therapist's discretion.

Outcomes:
• Dressing (Nottingham Stroke Dressing Assessment)
• Self-care (self-care section of Rivermead ADL Scale)
• Perceived health (Nottingham Health Profile) | Both groups improved significantly during treatment phase on all 3 measures. Neither group showed any change during nontreatment phase.

Group that received treatment first maintained its improvement at 6 months. | Lack of control for number of interventions (therapist determined amount of service to be provided to each participant) | Dressing practice for stroke patients is effective in improving independence in dressing, and improvements are maintained after therapy ends. |

Reference: Walker, M. F., Drummond, A. E. R., & Lincoln, N. B. (1996). Evaluation of dressing practice for stroke patients after discharge from hospital: A crossover design study. *Clinical Rehabilitation, 10,* 23–31.

(continued)

Evidence Table on Occupational Therapy and Adults With Stroke: Human Studies (continued)

Author/Year	Study Objectives	Level/Design/Participants	Intervention & Outcome Measures	Results	Study Limitations	Implications for OT
Walker et al. (1999)	Study effects of occupational therapy on stroke patients not admitted to hospital	I—Randomized controlled trial N = 185 (94 men, 91 women); 94 in experimental group, 91 in control group Average age: 74.3 years	Participants were randomly assigned to occupational therapy group or control group. Occupational therapy focused on active intervention to promote independence in ADLs and IADLs. Intervention, delivered by occupational therapists in participants' homes, occurred for up to 5 months. Frequency of treatment was determined by therapist, patient, and caregiver (average number of visits, 5.8; average length, 52 minutes). Control group received no treatment. Outcomes: • Instrumental ADLs (Extended ADL Scale) • ADLs (Barthel Index) • Motor performance (gross-function section of Rivermead Motor Assessment) • Strain on caregiver (Carer Strain Index) • Mood of patient and caregiver (General Health Questionnaire) • Handicap (London Handicap Scale)	Experimental group scored significantly higher than control group on Extended ADL Scale, Barthel Index, Carer Strain Index, and London Handicap Scale. Experimental group performed significantly better than control group on Rivermead Motor Assessment when comparison focused on subsets of scores.	Attention bias	Occupational therapy may reduce disability in stroke survivors not admitted to hospital.

Reference: Walker, M. F., Gladman, J. R., Lincoln, N. B., Siemonsma, P., & Whiteley, T. (1999). Occupational therapy for stroke patients not admitted to hospital: A randomised controlled trial. *Lancet, 354,* 278–280.

Walker et al. (2004)	Review evidence regarding efficacy of community occupational therapy for stroke patients	I—Systematic review (meta-analysis) of 8 randomized controlled trials *N* = 1,143 participants (602 men, 541 women) across 8 trials Average age: 71.4 years	Researchers reviewed randomized controlled trials using Cochrane Collaboration methodology. They focused on individual data rather than group data. Outcomes: • Extended ADLs (Nottingham Extended ADLs Scale [NEADL]) • Personal ADL (Barthel Index or Rivermead ADL Scale) • General health (General Health Questionnaire) • Leisure activity (Nottingham Leisure Questionnaire [NLQ]) • Death	Participants receiving occupational therapy had higher scores on NEADL and NLQ at end of intervention and end of trial than patients receiving usual care. Participants receiving occupational therapy that emphasized ADL had higher scores on NEADL and significant 29% reduction in odds of activity limitation (assessed using Barthel Index or Rivermead ADL) at end of intervention.	Study is of good quality.	Community occupational therapy contributes to higher levels of activity in stroke patients.

Reference: Walker, M. F., Leonardi-Bee, J., Bath, P., Langhorne, P., Dewey, M., Corr, S., et al. (2004). Individual patient data meta-analysis of randomized controlled trials of community occupational therapy for stroke patients. *Stroke, 35,* 2226–2232.

Wang et al. (2005)	Compare the effectiveness of neurodevelopmental treatment or Bobath with orthopedic treatment to improve balance and lower limb function in stroke survivors	I—Randomized controlled trial *N* = 44 (n = 21 with stroke with spasticity [11 in orthopedic, 10 in Bobath], n = 23 with stroke with relative recovery [12 in orthopedic, 11 in Bobath]) Participants were all rehabilitation inpatients at a medical center.	Neurodevelopmental treatment with an emphasis on retraining normal alignment and normal movement patterns based on Bobath concept: 40 minutes per session 5 tmes per week for a total of 20 sessions Control: Orthopedic treatment—passive, assistive, active, and progressive resistive exercise, 40 minutes per session, 5 times per week for a total of 20 sessions Outcomes: • Stroke Impairment Assessment Set (SIAS) • MAS • Berg Balance Scale (BBS) • Stroke Impact Scale (SIS)	For those with spasticity, there were improvements in both groups on the SIAS motor control of the lower extremity, MAS, and BBS. Those in the Bobath group had significantly better performance than the orthopedic group on the MAS, SIAS—tone, and SIS. For those with relative recovery, both groups demonstrated improved performance on the BBS and SIS. Those in the Bobath group performed significantly better than the orthopedic on both the BBS and SIS, in addition to the MAS.	Limitation of trial to 4 weeks may not be optimal. No long-term follow-up; follow-up limited to immediately following intervention period. The level of improvement exhibited by the Bobath group may have been skewed by an initial difference in function between the two groups as demonstrated by MAS and BBS scores.	This study provides support for efficacy of Bobath intervention for improving balance and lower-limb function in stroke survivors.

Reference: Wang, R. Y., Chen, H. I., Chen, C. Y., & Yang, Y. R. (2005). Efficacy of Bobath versus orthopaedic approach on impairment and function at different motor recovery stages after stroke. *Clinical Rehabilitation, 19,* 155–164.

(continued)

Evidence Table on Occupational Therapy and Adults With Stroke: Human Studies *(continued)*

Author/Year	Study Objectives	Level/Design/Participants	Intervention & Outcome Measures	Results	Study Limitations	Implications for OT
Winstein et al. (2004)	Evaluate effects of 2 treatment approaches immediately following treatment and 9 months after stroke	I—Randomized controlled trial $N = 60$ (33 men, 27 women); 20 per group Average age: Not reported; only 3 participants younger than 35 or older than 75 years	Participants were stratified by severity (using Orpington Prognostic Scale), then randomly assigned to standard care, task-specific functional training (involving pointing, grasping, and stirring) plus standard care, or strengthening and motor control (using resistance) plus standard care. Standard care was delivered by occupational therapists, experimental treatments by physical therapists, in rehabilitation hospital. Experimental treatments occurred in 1-hour sessions 5 days per week for 4–6 weeks. Outcomes: • Range of motion, pain, sensory perception, and motor function (upper-extremity portion of FMA) • Isometric torque at shoulder, elbow, and wrist (sum of distances from joint center to dynamometer placement for each joint) • Grip and pinch strength • Function (Functional Test of Hemiparetic Upper Extremity [FTHUE]) • Self-care and mobility (FIM)	Immediately following treatment, participants in experimental groups showed significantly greater improvements in motor function and isometric torque than participants receiving standard care alone. Participants in experimental groups with less severe stroke showed significantly greater improvements in motor function, isometric torque, and FTHUE scores than counterparts receiving standard care alone. At 9 months, participants in functional training group with less severe stroke showed significantly greater improvements in isometric torque than counterparts in strength training group.	Possible bias from evaluator not being blinded to group assignment	Task-specific therapy is effective in improving motor function after stroke, especially with patients demonstrating less severe impairments.

Reference: Winstein, C. J., Rose, D. K., Tan, S. M., Lewthwaite, R., Chui, H. C., & Azen, S. P. (2004). A randomized controlled comparison of upper-extremity rehabilitation strategies in acute stroke: A pilot study of immediate and long-term outcomes. *Archives of Physical Medicine and Rehabilitation, 85,* 620–628.

Author (Year)	Study Design / Participants	Intervention / Outcomes	Results	Comments
Wittenberg et al. (2003)	Compare effects of CIMT and less-intensive intervention on motor function and brain physiology in stroke patients 1 year or more after stroke I—Randomized controlled trial N = 16 (13 men, 3 women); 9 in experimental group, 7 in control group Average age: 64.0 years	Participants were randomly assigned to receive CIMT or control therapy. CIMT involved restraint of unaffected upper extremity during waking hours and task-oriented therapy with affected upper extremity. Control therapy involved task performance on unaffected side. CIMT, delivered in clinical center, occurred 6 hours per day for 8 days, 4 hours per day for 2 days (1 weekend). Control therapy, also delivered in clinical center, occurred 3 hours per day for 8 days. Participants rested on weekend. Outcomes: • Motor function (WMFT) • Function during daily activities (MAL) • ADLs (AMPS) • Changes in motor cortex (TMS) • Changes in motor task–related activation (positron emission tomography)	Experimental group performed significantly better than control group on MAL but not on AMPS and WMFT. TMS-center of gravity of map of unaffected side shifted significantly in both groups in medial direction. Difference between groups was not significant. TMS-map volume ratio (map volume of affected side divided by map volume of unaffected side) increased more in experimental group than in control group, and difference approached significance. Paired-pulse facilitation on unaffected side increased significantly more in experimental group than in control group. Motor cortical activation on affected side decreased (improved) more in experimental group than in control group.	Study is of good quality. Measurable physiological changes may accompany rehabilitation interventions emphasizing practice.

Reference: Wittenberg, G. F., Chen, R., Ishii, K., Bushara, K. O., Eckloff, S., Croarkin, E., et al. (2003). Constraint-induced therapy in stroke: Magnetic-stimulation motor maps and cerebral activation. *Neurorehabilitation and Neural Repair, 17,* 48–57.

Author (Year)	Study Design / Participants	Intervention	Results	Comments
Wolf et al. (2006)	Compare effects of 2-week multisite program of CIMT and usual and customary care for patients in subacute phase of stroke (3–9 months since occurrence) I—Randomized controlled trial N = 222 (142 men, 80 women); 106 in experimental group, 116 in control group Average age: 62.2 years	Participants were randomly assigned to a group receiving constraint-induced movement therapy (experimental group) or a group receiving usual and customary care (control group). Experimental group received therapy 6 hours per day for 10 weekdays and were encouraged to wear a mitt on the unaffected hand for a target of 90% of	Immediately following treatment, experimental group showed significantly larger improvements than control group in quality and speed of arm movement, and except on 2 motor-function strength items, and in quality and amount of real-world arm use.	Possible bias from difference between groups in intensity of treatment CIMT produces improvements in patients in subacute phase of stroke. These improvements persist for at least 1 year.

(continued)

Author/Year	Study Objectives	Level/Design/Participants	Intervention & Outcome Measures	Results	Study Limitations	Implications for OT
			waking hours on those 10 days and related weekends. Therapy involved both shaping and repetitive-task training. Control group received care ranging from no treatment to use of orthotics to various occupational and physical therapy approaches. Outcomes: • Quality and speed of arm movement (WMFT) • Quality and amount of real-world arm use (MAL)	At 4-, 8-, and 12-month follow-ups, experimental group showed significantly greater improvements in speed of arm movement and in quality and amount of real-world arm use.		

Reference: Wolf, S. L., Winstein, C. J., Miller, J. P., Taub, E., Uswatte, G., Morris, D., et al. (2006). Effect of constraint-induced movement therapy on upper extremity function 3 to 9 months after stroke: The EXCITE randomized clinical trial. *JAMA, 296,* 2095–2104.

Author/Year	Study Objectives	Level/Design/Participants	Intervention & Outcome Measures	Results	Study Limitations	Implications for OT
Woodford & Price (2007)	Determine the effectiveness of electromyographic biofeedback (EMG-BFB) to improve motor recovery following stroke	I—Systematic review Thirteen randomized and nonrandomized controlled trials with 269 participants were included in the review	Trials comparing EMG-BFB with control for motor recovery; all trials compared EMG-BFB plus standard physical therapy either alone or with sham EMG-BFB. Outcomes: *Primary*—Change in muscle power *Secondary*—Range of motion, gait, functional ability, proportion of participants with muscle weakness	The results of the studies were mixed. Benefit from EMG-BFB was noted for range of motion of the shoulder but not for ankle, wrist, or knee joints. One study using a motor assessment scale noted a significant improvement for those with EMG-BFB. No improvement was noted for stride length or gait speed. Two studies using similar assessment scales to measure functional outcomes noted a beneficial effect of EMG-BFB.	Overall, trials had limited number of participants, were not well designed, and used a wide range of outcome measures.	There is limited evidence to support or refute the effectiveness of biofeedback in enhancing motor function after stroke.

Reference: Woodford, H., & Price, C. (2007). EMG biofeedback for the recovery of motor function after stroke. *Cochrane Database of Systematic Reviews,* Issue No. 2., Art. No. CD004585.

	Purpose	Design/Sample	Intervention	Results	Follow-Up	Implications
Wu et al. (2007)	Assess the benefits of mCIMT on motor function, daily function, and health-related quality of life (HRQL) in elderly stroke survivors.	I—Randomized controlled trial 26 elderly patients with stroke (mean = 72 years) who met motor criteria for participation (n = 13 mCIMT, n = 13 traditional rehabilitation)	Participants were randomly assigned to mCIMT or control groups. Participants in both groups received individualized 2-hour occupational therapy sessions, 5 times per week for 3 weeks. For mCIMT participants, therapy consisted of shaping and adaptive, repetitive task practice techniques, with 15 minutes of therapy time spent on reducing abnormal muscle tone when needed. In addition, participants wore mitts on the less-affected hand every weekday for 6 hours during a time of frequent arm use. For control group participants, therapy consisted of approximately 75% traditional rehabilitation focused on neurodevelopmental technique and 25% training in compensatory techniques using the unaffected limb to perform functional tasks. Outcomes: • FMA • FIM • MAL • SIS	Compared with controls, the mCIMT group showed significantly greater gains on FMA, FIM, MAL, and SIS scores when assessed immediately posttreatment.	No follow-up assessments were made to assess long-term effects.	Elderly stroke survivors, who may tolerate the demands of mCIMT better than standard CIMT, benefit from a modified CIMT program during inpatient rehabilitation.

Reference: Wu, C. Y., Chen, C. L., Tsai, W. C., Lin, K. C., & Chou, S. H. (2007). A randomized controlled trial of modified constraint-induced movement therapy for elderly stroke survivors: Changes in motor impairment, daily functioning, and quality of life. *Archives of Physical Medicine and Rehabilitation, 88*, 273–278.

	Purpose	Design/Sample	Intervention	Results	Follow-Up	Implications
Wu et al. (2007)	Use motion analysis technology to compare motor control during functional reach in patients who participated in mCIMT with patients who participated in traditional rehabilitation	I—Randomized controlled trial 30 patients with stroke who meet motor criteria for participation in mCIMT (n = 15 mCIMT, n = 15 traditional rehabilitation [TR])	Participants were randomly assigned to mCIMT or control group. Participants in both groups received individualized 2-hour occupational therapy sessions, 5 times per week for 3 weeks. For mCIMT participants, therapy consisted of shaping and adap-	Analysis of covariance revealed significantly greater improvements for the mCIMT group in temporal, spatial, and preplanning measures generated by kinematic analysis, but more so when performing the bilateral task. The mCIMT	No follow-up assessments were made to assess long-term effects.	In addition to its impact on functional outcomes, mCIMT also results in improved quality of movement during arm reach, as measured with motion analysis technology.

(continued)

Evidence Table on Occupational Therapy and Adults With Stroke: Human Studies *(continued)*

Author/Year	Study Objectives	Level/Design/Participants	Intervention & Outcome Measures	Results	Study Limitations	Implications for OT
			tive, repetitive task practice techniques, with 15 minutes of therapy time spent on reducing abnormal muscle tone when needed. In addition, participants wore mitts on the less-affected hand every weekday for 6 hours during a time of frequent arm use. TR group members received neurodevelopmental treatments at the same dosage. Outcomes: • Kinematic analysis of spatial and temporal movement efficiency and type of movement control during unilateral (reaching forward to depress a bell) and bilateral (opening a drawer and reaching inside to retrieve an eyeglass case) tasks • MAL • FIM Outcomes were assessed immediately after the 3-week intervention.	improvements on MAL and FIM were also significantly greater than the control group.		

Reference: Wu, C. Y., Lin, K.-C., Chen, H. C., Chen, I. H., & Hong, W. H. (2007). Effects of modified constraint-induced movement therapy on movement kinematics and daily function in patients with stroke: A kinematic study of motor control mechanisms. *Neurorehabilitation and Neural Repair, 21,* 460–466.

Author/Year	Study Objectives	Level/Design/Participants	Intervention & Outcome Measures	Results	Study Limitations	Implications for OT
Wu et al. (1998)	Investigate how object affordances (physical properties) affect reaching performance in stroke patients	I—Randomized controlled trial; counterbalanced repeated-measures design *N* = 38 (16 men, 22 women); 14 stroke patients (9 men, 5 women), 24 people without disability (7 men, 17 women; control group) Average age: 62.7 years	Participants were randomly assigned to AB or BA sequence of conditions. Condition A, enriched, involved participants reaching forward to a chopper and pushing down handle to chop a mushroom. Condition B, impoverished, involved participants reaching forward to a disguised chopper with nothing in it and pushing down handle. All participants performed 10 trials per condition within 1 day.	Participants showed significantly better organization of reaching movement in enriched condition on 3 measures (movement time, total displacement, and number of movement units) and marginally significant effect on 1 measure (percentage of reach where peak velocity occurs).	Possible bias from experimenters' expectations	Occupational therapists might provide natural objects for completing tasks and functional information on objects to enhance stroke patients' functional performance.

Occupational therapist delivered intervention in laboratory.

Outcomes:
- Movement organization (movement time)
- Total displacement, or length of path of hand in three-dimensional space
- Number of movement units, indication of smoothness of movement (combination of 1 acceleration phase and 1 deceleration phase)
- Percentage of reach where peak velocity occurs, indication of control strategy (proportion of reach corresponding to changeover from aceleration to deceleration)
- Amplitude of peak velocity, overall indication of force of movement (highest level of velocity achieved during reach)

Reference: Wu, C., Trombly, C. A., Lin, K., & Tickle-Degnen, L. (1998). Effects of object affordances on reaching performance in persons with and without cerebrovascular accident. *American Journal of Occupational Therapy, 52*, 179–187.

| Wu et al. (2000) | Examine effects of context on reaching performance in stroke patients and persons without disability | I—Randomized controlled trial; counterbalanced repeated-measures design *N* = 39; 14 stroke patients (9 men, 5 women), 25 persons without disability (8 men, 17 women; control group) Average age: 63.1 years | Participants were randomly assigned to AB or BA sequence of conditions. Condition A, enriched, involved reaching forward to scoop coins off table. Condition B, impoverished, involved reaching forward to perform the same motion without coins present. Participants performed 10 trials per condition within 1 day. Occupational therapist presented conditions in laboratory. Outcomes: • Speed (movement time) • Directness (total displacement) • Smoothness (movement units) | Participants with stroke showed significantly faster, more direct, more pre-planned, and smoother movements under enriched condition than under impoverished condition. Persons without disability showed significantly faster, more direct, and more pre-planned movements under enriched condition and had nearly significant results for smoothness. Between groups and across both conditions, persons | Study is of good quality. | Functional motor training of stroke patients should use enriched affordances that include natural objects. |

(continued)

Evidence Table on Occupational Therapy and Adults With Stroke: Human Studies (continued)

Author/Year	Study Objectives	Level/Design/Participants	Intervention & Outcome Measures	Results	Study Limitations	Implications for OT
			• Planning strategy (percentage of reach where peak velocity occurs) • Force (peak velocity)	without disability showed significantly faster, more direct, more preplanned, more forceful, and smoother movements than stroke patients.		

Reference: Wu, C., Trombly, C. A., Lin, K., & Tickle-Degnen, L. (2000). A kinematic study of contextual effects on reaching performance in persons with and without stroke: Influences of object availability. *Archives of Physical Medicine and Rehabilitation, 81*, 95–101.

Author/Year	Study Objectives	Level/Design/Participants	Intervention & Outcome Measures	Results	Study Limitations	Implications for OT
Young et al. (1983)	Examine effects of pairing cancellation and visual-scanning training with block-design training in remediation of perceptual problems of stroke patients with left hemiplegia	II—Nonrandomized controlled trial *N* = 27 (gender not reported); 9 per group Average age: 64.0 years	Participants were divided into 3 groups of 9 matched for age, education, time since onset of stroke, and degree of deficit. Group 1 received 1 hour of routine occupational therapy (ADLs and perceptual tasks). Group 2 received 20 minutes of training in routine occupational therapy (as in Group 1), 20 minutes of training in cancellation, and 20 minutes of training in visual scanning. Group 3 received 20 minutes of training in cancellation, 20 minutes of training in visual scanning, and 20 minutes of training in block design. Training was delivered by occupational therapist in clinic 1 hour per day for 20 successive weekdays. Outcomes: • Cognitive performance (Digit Symbol, Picture Completion, Block Design, Picture Arrangement, and Object Assembly subtests of Wechsler Adult Intelligence Scale) • Perceptual processing (letter-cancellation task, Reading subtest of Wide Range Achievement Test, ability to copy address, and ability to count faces)	Groups 2 and 3 improved significantly more on measures of visual scanning, reading, and writing than Group 1 did. Group 3 improved significantly more on same measures than Group 2 did.	Possible bias from therapists' expectations and lack of randomization	Interventions that emphasize training in cancellation, visual scanning, and block design might improve perceptual performance of stroke patients with left hemiplegia.

Reference: Young, G. C., Collins, D., & Hren, M. (1983). Effect of pairing scanning training with block design training in the remediation of perceptual problems in left hemiplegics. *Journal of Clinical Neuropsychology, 5*, 201–212.

| Zinn et al. (2004) | Determine effect of cognitive impairment on stroke patients' access to and quality of rehabilitation services and on their functional outcomes | II—Cohort study

$N = 272$ (264 men, 8 women); 185 with cognitive impairment, 87 without

Average age: 67.1 years | Participants were stroke patients at 11 Department of Veterans Affairs medical centers. On admission, they were assessed for whether or not they had cognitive impairment. They were followed for 6 months after stroke.

Outcomes:
- Quality of rehabilitation services
- Timing of rehabilitation services (days from onset to acute care, length of stay in acute care, and time to initiation of postacute care)
- Receipt of rehabilitation services
- Frequency of receipt of cognition-related components of care (e.g., occupational therapy evaluations)
- Frequency of evaluations for depression
- Frequency of evaluations for speech therapy, cognition, and communication and social functioning disorders, and of brain scans and magnetic resonance imaging
- Discharge destination
- ADLs (motor score on Functional Independence Measure)
- Instrumental ADLs (Lawton IADLs) | Participants with cognitive impairment had significantly longer lengths of stay in acute care than participants without cognitive impairment; significantly more were still receiving rehabilitation at 6 months.

Significantly more participants with cognitive impairment had cognitive goals in their treatment plans.

Controlling for baseline function and rehabilitation process, participants with cognitive impairment performed significantly worse on IADLs than participants without impairment. | Possible bias from exclusion of patients who could not follow 2-step command, variability of services across settings, and patient population (veterans, mostly men) | Improved diagnosis and targeted provision of appropriate services might improve outcomes for stroke patients with cognitive impairment. |

Reference: Zinn, S., Dudley, T. K., Bosworth, H. B., Hoenig, H. M., Duncan, P. W., & Horner, R. D. (2004). The effect of poststroke cognitive impairment on rehabilitation process and functional outcome. *Archives of Physical Medicine and Rehabilitation, 85,* 1084–1090.

Evidence Table on Occupational Therapy and Adults With Stroke: Level V Human Studies

Author/Year	Study Objectives	Level/Design/Participants	Intervention & Outcome Measures	Results	Study Limitations	Implications for OT
Calautti & Baron (2003)	Review literature on motor activation studies of stroke patients performed with positron emission tomography (PET) and functional magnetic resonance imaging (fMRI)	V—Review of literature 20 studies, 117 references	Researchers reviewed studies published from 1991 through 2002 using PET or fMRI with stroke patients who had experienced cortical or subcortical strokes and had recovered or were still recovering from motor deficits. Studies encompassed were cross-sectional or longitudinal.	A damaged adult brain can reorganize to compensate for motor deficits. The main mechanism to recover motor ability is enhanced activity in preexisting networks, including disconnected motor cortex after subcortical stroke and infarct rim after cortical stroke. Involvement of non-motor and contralesional motor areas has been consistently reported. The emerging belief is that the greater the involvement of ipsilesional motor network, the better the recovery. This hypothesis is supported by enhanced activity of ipsilesional primary motor cortex induced by motor training and acute pharmacological interventions, in parallel with improved motor function.	Caution is advisable in interpreting results of Level V reviews because the reviews do not include information on databases searched and inclusion and exclusion criteria.	Rehabilitative interventions that can reactivate physiological motor network should enhance motor recovery. Motor-training procedures can influence motor network reorganization, and training-induced brain plasticity is possible not only in subacute, but also in chronic, stroke survivors. Clinical significance of other findings is not yet clear.

Reference: Calautti, C., & Baron, J. C. (2003). Functional neuroimaging studies of motor recovery after stroke in adults: A review. *Stroke, 34,* 1553–1556.

Dancause (2006)	Review the evidence for cognitive reorganization with specific emphasis on nonhuman primate studies and stroke	V—Review of literature 171 references	Describe the remodeling of representational maps of the forelimb and plasticity with specific emphasis on nonhuman primate studies and stroke	A review of the literature indicates that learning and practice result in adaptive plasticity. A proposed mechanism includes the reinforcement of existing (albeit secondary or alternative neuronal) circuits through a potential release of inhibition that would result in the activation of previously latent connection between two neurons. In addition, sprouting or formation of new polysynaptic connections is also proposed.	Caution is advisable in interpreting results of Level V reviews because the reviews do not include information on databases searched and inclusion and exclusion criteria.	There is considerable neuroscience support for the mammalian brain's capacity to reorganize after experimental lesions or cerebrovascular accident.

Reference: Dancause, N. (2006). Neurophysiological and anatomical plasticity in the adult sensorimotor cortex. *Reviews in the Neurosciences, 17,* 561–580.

| Johansson (2003) | Review literature on extent to which post-ischemic events can influence lesion-induced plasticity | V—Review of literature
70 references | Researcher reviewed studies of environmental effects on (1) intact and lesioned brain, (2) neuronal and dendritic morphology and dendritic spines, and (4) lesion-induced progenitor cell differentiation. He also reviewed studies comparing effects of environmental enrichment, social interaction, and physical activity and studies examining the interaction of the environment with neocortical transplantation and drugs. | Environmental enrichment following ischemia significantly improves functional outcomes, increases dendrite branching and number of dendritic spines in contralateral cortex, influences expression of many genes, and modifies lesion-induced stem cell differentiation in the hippocampus. Further, environmental factors can interact with specific interventions such as necrotic grafting and drug treatment. | Caution is advisable in interpreting results of Level V reviews because the reviews do not include information on databases searched and inclusion and exclusion criteria. | In evaluating clinical applicability of animal studies, occupational therapists should take into account that animals' environments often provide no stimulation. |

Reference: Johansson, B. B. (2003). Environmental influence on recovery after brain lesions: Experimental and clinical data. *Journal of Rehabilitation Medicine, 41*(Suppl.), 11–16.

| Nudo (2003) | Review literature on restoration of function long after stroke | V—Review of literature
54 references | Researcher reviewed studies on skill-dependent plasticity in uninjured motor cortex and on adaptive plasticity in injured brains. | Sensorimotor learning and cortical injury interact. Following injury, person's sensorimotor experience shapes structure and function of undamaged parts. | Caution is advisable in interpreting results of Level V reviews because the reviews do not include information on databases searched and inclusion and exclusion criteria. | New rehabilitative interventions using therapy and/or drugs may modulate neuroplasticity. |

Reference: Nudo, R. J., (2003). Functional and structural plasticity in motor cortex: Implications for stroke recovery. *Physical Medicine and Physical Rehabilitation Clinics of North America. 14,* S57–S76.

| Patten et al. (2004) | Review literature on phenomenon of weakness in stroke patients with hemiplegia, review literature identifying physiological substrates of weakness, and review literature on strength training (progressive resistance training) for functional improvement | V—Review of literature
111 references | Researchers reviewed literature on distribution, functional consequences, and mechanisms of weakness in stroke patients with hemiplegia, and possibility of counteracting weakness. | Effortful activity and strength training do not exacerbate spasticity, per se. Impaired strength may play a prominent role in compromising functional performance. Strength training produces positive effects on various indices of functional outcome, such as gait speed, stair-climbing ability, and ADLs. Functional effects appear to be persistent. | Caution is advisable in interpreting results of Level V reviews because the reviews do not include information on databases searched and inclusion and exclusion criteria. | Strength training has a role in reversing weakness in stroke patients with hemiplegia—as an adjunct to or augmentation of traditional rehabilitation, not as a replacement for it. |

Reference: Patten, C., Lexell, J., & Brown, H. E. (2004). Weakness and strength training in persons with poststroke hemiplegia: Rationale, method, and efficacy. *Journal of Rehabilitation Research & Development, 41,* 293–312.

(continued)

Author/Year	Study Objectives	Level/Design/Participants	Intervention & Outcome Measures	Results	Study Limitations	Implications for OT
Rossini et al. (2007)	Review the results of neuroimaging experimental studies on brain plasticity following stroke	V—Review of literature 156 references	To examine the evidence related to a variety of mechanisms following environmental inputs after a lesion: synaptogenesis; dendritic arborization; recruitment of pathways that are functionally homologous to, but anatomically distinct from, damaged ones; and reinforcement of existing but functionally silent synaptic connections.	Evidence indicates that neuronal aggregates that are adjacent to or distant from a lesion in the sensorimotor area can adopt the function of the injured area. Results from imaging studies indicate that recovery of motor function following a stroke is associated with a progressive change of activation patterns in specific brain structures.	Caution is advisable in interpreting results of Level V reviews because the reviews do not include information on databases searched and inclusion and exclusion criteria.	There is considerable neuroscience support for the human brain's capacity to reorganize with functional recovery after stroke.

Reference: Rossini, P. M., Altamura, C., Ferreri, F., Melgari, J. M., Tecchio, F., Tombini, M., et al. (2007). Neuroimaging experimental studies on brain plasticity in recovery from stroke. *Europa Medicophysiology, 43*, 241–254.

Woldag & Hummelsheim (2002)	Review literature on evidenced-based strategies for motor rehabilitation in stroke patients	V—Review of literature 42 references	Researchers reviewed literature on physiotherapeutic approaches, repetitive motor activity, electrical muscle stimulation initiated by electromyography (EMG), role of sensorimotor coupling, motor imagery and repeated mental practice, and motor training in natural context.	Bobath approach, proprioceptive neuromuscular facilitation, and Brunnstrom approach are alike in effect on recovery of motor function. Task-specific "motor relearning program" may be more effective than rehabilitation strategies that adhere exclusively to Bobath approach. Repetitive movement greatly benefits functional outcome of motor rehabilitation of centrally paretic arm and hand. EMG-initiated electrical muscle stimulation produces results similar to those of repetitive movement, provided that movements are initiated repetitively.	Caution is advisable in interpreting results of Level V reviews because the reviews do not include information on databases searched and inclusion and exclusion criteria.	Repetitive motor practice (including EMG-initiated electrical muscle stimulation) and motor activity in natural context both are favorable for motor recovery. Among approaches involving motor activity in natural context, constraint-induced movement therapy appears to be useful and is strongly recommended.

Motor imagery and repeated mental practice produce representational modifications in the brain that are comparable to those induced by physical practice. However, benefits are not superior to those of active motor training.

Forced use of affected extremities in natural context (as in constraint-induced movement therapy) produces significant benefits in motor function.

Reference: Woldag, H., & Hummelsheim, H. (2002). Evidence-based physiotherapeutic concepts for improving arm and hand function in stroke patients: A review. *Journal of Neurology, 249,* 518–528.

| Wolf et al. (2002) | Review concept of CIMT and analyze existing data on its use in helping stroke patients overcome upper extremity impairments | V—Review of literature 22 studies | Researchers reviewed literature on CIMT and critically analyzed available studies. | Data are encouraging. Appropriate population may be patients with adequate balance and safety while wearing restraint and ability to initiate at least 20° of wrist extension and at least 10° of extension of 2 digits in addition to first digit of affected hand. Success may depend on cooperation from patient and intense repetitive use through practice and shaping. | Possible bias from studies included in review being primarily uncontrolled trials or small controlled ones | CIMT has promise for helping selected stroke patients improve upper extremity function. Task novelty and challenge seem to be important to recovery of function. |

Reference: Wolf, S. L., Blanton, S., Baer, H., Breshears, J., & Butler, A. J. (2002). Repetitive task practice: A critical review of constraint-induced movement therapy in stroke. *Neurologist, 8,* 325–338.

Appendix C.
Selected *CPT*™ Coding for Occupational Therapy Evaluations and Interventions

The following chart is a guide to assist in making clinically appropriate decisions in selecting the most relevant *Current Procedural Terminology™ (CPT)* code to describe occupation therapy evaluation and intervention. Occupational therapy practitioners should use the most appropriate code from the current *CPT* based on specific services provided, individual patient goals, payer policy, and common usage.

Examples of Occupational Therapy Evaluation and Intervention	Suggested *CPT* Code(s)
• Provide instruction and training in compensatory techniques for performing daily self-care activities • Assist patient in incorporating energy conservation techniques to facilitate participation in instrumental activities of daily living (IADLs) • Provide training in use of environmental controls and adaptive equipment to assure safe, independent living within the home environment	97535—Self-care/home management training (e.g., activities of daily living [ADLs] and compensatory training, meal preparation, safety procedures, instructions in use of assistive technology devices/adaptive equipment), direct (one-on-one) contact by the provider, each 15 minutes
• Assess patient requirements for specialized mobility equipment, such as powered wheelchairs, to enable community and work participation • Provide recommendations for wheelchair modifications to ensure optimal sitting posture in order to maintain skin integrity, prevent pressure sores, and facilitate performance in ADLs and IADLs	97542—Wheelchair management (e.g., assessment, fitting, training), each 15 minutes
• Evaluate/assess changes in such areas as – Neuromusculoskeletal and movement-related functions, presence of movement dysfunction (e.g., tremor, spasticity, flaccidity, rigidity, bradykinesia, ataxia, dyskinesia, athetosis) – Sensory functions and pain – Mental functions, depression, denial, anxiety about the progressive nature of the disease	97003—Occupational therapy evaluation 97004—Occupational therapy reevaluation 97750—Physical performance test or measurement (e.g., musculoskeletal, functional capacity), with written report, each 15 minutes
• Provide functional exercises to increase range of motion, strength, and mobility to enable increased participation in daily activities	97110—Therapeutic procedure, one or more areas, each 15 minutes; therapeutic exercises to develop strength and endurance, range of motion, and flexibility 97113—Therapeutic procedure, one or more areas, each 15 minutes; aquatic therapy with therapeutic exercises

(continued)

Examples of Occupational Therapy Evaluation and Intervention	Suggested CPT Code(s)
• Design graded tasks to increase coordination and balance • Provide training in proper use of adaptive equipment to assist with balance and facilitate community mobility	97112—Therapeutic procedure, one or more areas, each 15 minutes; neuromuscular reeducation of movement, balance, coordination, kinesthetic sense, posture, and/or proprioception for sitting and/or standing activities
• Administer the Rivermead Behavioural Memory Test to determine extent of memory impairments in everyday activities and the need for occupational therapy intervention related to cognitive skills	96125—Standardized cognitive performance testing (e.g., Ross Information Processing Assessment) per hour of a qualified health professional's time, both face-to-face time administering tests to the patient and time interpreting these test results and preparing the report
• Train in use of memory exercises to enhance the ability to remember telephone numbers and e-mail addresses while at home or work • Develop strategies to ensure completion of morning routine, such as medication management, safely preparing breakfast and school lunches, and organizing daily schedule for completion of household activities	97532—Development of cognitive skills to improve attention, memory, problem solving (includes compensatory training), direct (one-on-one) patient contact by the provider, each 15 minutes
• Provide occupation-based activities to increase ability to perform avocational or work tasks	97530—Therapeutic activities, direct (one-on-one) patient contact by the provider (use of dynamic activities to improve functional performance), each 15 minutes
• Assess body structure and body functions that influence feeding and eating, environmental influence, positioning, and physical and cognitive problems that affect feeding, eating, and swallowing	92610, 92611, 92612—Clinical evaluation of swallowing function (see CPT for precise descriptions of possible tests)
• Train in the use of compensatory strategies, appropriate positioning, adaptive equipment, and food textures to maximize oral intake and nutritional status	92526—Treatment of swallowing dysfunction and/or oral function for feeding
• Teach energy conservation techniques to facilitate increased community participation • Analyze client routines and train in modifying/changing daily routines, roles, and habits to reintegrate client into independent shopping, work, or volunteer activities	92537—Community/work reintegration training (e.g., shopping, transportation, money management, avocational activities or work environment/modification analysis, work task analysis, use of assistive technology device/adaptive equipment), direct one-on-one contact by the provider, each 15 minutes
• Assess and design an orthotic to support the wrist to overcome weakness and allow client to maintain hand in proper position to carry out daily activities • Prevent loss of range of motion by providing hand and foot drop splints [Refer to Medicare National Level II HCPCS Codes, available at www.cms.hhs.gov/hcpcsreleasecodesets/, for billing actual orthosis]	97760—Orthotic(s) management and training (including assessment and fitting when not otherwise reported), upper extremity(s), lower extremity(s) and/or trunk, each 15 minutes 97762—Checkout for orthotic/prosthetic use, established patient, each 15 minutes
• Provide joint mobilization to the wrist and fingers to maintain joint play and joint integrity in order to grasp utensils and other items such as pens and toothbrush	97140—Manual therapy techniques (e.g., mobilization/manipulation, manual lymphatic drainage, manual traction), one or more regions, each 15 minutes

Reference: American Medial Association. (2007). *CPT* 2008. Chicago: Author.

Notes: The *CPT 2008* codes referenced in this document do not represent all of the possible codes that may be used in occupational therapy evaluation and intervention. Not all payers will reimburse for all codes. Refer to *CPT 2008* for the complete list of available codes.

CPT™ is a trademark of the American Medical Association (AMA). *CPT* five-digit codes, nomenclature, and other data are copyright © 2007 by the American Medical Association. All Rights Reserved. Reprinted with permission. No fee schedules, basic units, relative values, or related listings are included in *CPT*. The AMA assumes no liability for the data contained herein.

Codes shown refer to *CPT 2008*. *CPT* codes are updated annually. New and revised codes become effective January 1. Always refer to annual updated *CPT* publication for most current codes.

Appendix D.
2008 Selected *ICD-9-CM* Codes

430	Subarachnoid hemorrhage +
431	Intracerebral hemorrhage
432.0	Nontraumatic extradural hemorrhage
432.1	Subdural hemorrhage
433	Occlusion and stenosis of precerebral arteries +
433.0	Occlusion and stenosis of precerebral arteries, Basilar artery +
433.1	Occlusion and stenosis of precerebral arteries, Carotid artery +
433.2	Occlusion and stenosis of precerebral arteries, Vertebral artery +
434	Occlusion of cerebral arteries +
438	Late effects of cerebrovascular disease +
438.0	Late effects of cerebrovascular disease, Cognitive deficits
438.21	Late effects of cerebrovascular disease, Hemiplegia/hemiparesis, Hemiplegia affecting dominant side
438.22	Late effects of cerebrovascular disease, Hemiplegia/hemiparesis, Hemiplegia affecting nondominant side
438.31	Late effects of cerebrovascular disease, Monoplegia of upper limb, Monoplegia of upper limb affecting dominant side
438.32	Late effects of cerebrovascular disease, Monoplegia of upper limb, Monoplegia of upper limb affecting nondominant side
438.7	Late effects of cerebrovascular disease, Disturbance of vision
438.8	Late effects of cerebrovascular disease, Other late effects of cerebrovascular disease
438.81	Late effects of cerebrovascular disease, Other late effects of cerebrovascular disease, Apraxia
438.82	Late effects of cerebrovascular disease, Other late effects of cerebrovascular disease, Dysphagia
438.83	Late effects of cerebrovascular disease, Other late effects of cerebrovascular disease, Facial weakness
438.84	Late effects of cerebrovascular disease, Other late effects of cerebrovascular disease, Ataxia
438.85	Late effects of cerebrovascular disease, Other late effects of cerebrovascular disease, Vertigo

+ Codes that require an additional 4th and/or 5th digit to be coded correctly

Notes: Practitioners should use codes that most accurately reflect a patient's condition and diagnosis. For example, with the patient who has vertigo following a stroke, one should start with 438 (Late effects of cerebrovascular disease), then find the most descriptive term for the next digit, which is 438.8 (Other late effects of cerebrovascular disease), followed by the next most descriptive term, which is 438.85 for Vertigo. Thus, 438.85 is the most appropriate and accurate code for this patient, rather than the non-specific code 780.4, which describes only the symptom.

The *ICD-9-CM* 2008 codes referenced in this document do not represent all of the possible codes that may be used in occupational therapy evaluation and intervention. Refer to *ICD-9-CM* 2008 for the complete list of available codes.

For additional information, see http://www.cms.hhs.gov/ICD9ProviderDiagnosticCodes.

Reference: American Medical Association. (2008). *International classification of diseases, ninth revision, clinical modification* (ICD-9-CM 2008): *Hospital* (Vols. 1–3). Chicago: Author.

References

Abreu, B. C. (1994). *The quadraphonic approach: Evaluation and treatment of the brain-injured patient.* New York: Therapeutic Service Systems.

Ada, L., Foongchomcheay, A., & Canning, C. (2005). Supportive devices for preventing and treating subluxation of the shoulder after stroke. *Cochrane Database of Systematic Reviews,* Issue No. 1, Art. No. CD003863.

Aisen, M. L., Krebs, H. I., Hogan, N., McDowell, F., & Volpe, B. T. (1997). The effect of robot-assisted therapy and rehabilitative training on motor recovery following stroke. *Archives of Neurology, 54,* 443–446.

American Heart Association/American Stroke Association. (2007). *Heart disease and stroke statistics—2007 update.* Dallas, TX: American Heart Association.

American Medical Association. (2007). *CPT 2008.* Chicago: Author.

American Medical Association. (2008). *International classification of diseases, ninth revision, clinical modification* (ICD-9-CM 2008): Hospital (Vols. 1–3). Chicago: Author.

American National Standards Institute. (2003). ICC/ANSI A117. 1-2003 *Standard on accessible and usable buildings and facilities.* Washington, DC: Author.

American Occupational Therapy Association. (1979). Uniform terminology for occupational therapy. *Occupational Therapy News, 35*(11), 1–8.

American Occupational Therapy Association. (1989). Uniform terminology for occupational therapy (2nd ed.). *American Journal of Occupational Therapy, 43,* 808–815.

American Occupational Therapy Association. (1994). Uniform terminology for occupational therapy (3rd ed.). *American Journal of Occupational Therapy, 48,* 1047–1054.

American Occupational Therapy Association. (2004). Guidelines for supervision, roles, and responsibilities during the delivery of therapy services. *American Journal of Occupational Therapy, 58,* 663–667.

American Occupational Therapy Association. (2005). Standards of practice for occupational therapy. *American Journal of Occupational Therapy, 59,* 663–665.

American Occupational Therapy Association. (2006). Policy 1.44: Categories of occupational therapy personnel. In *Policy manual* (2007 ed., pp. 33–34). Bethesda, MD: Author.

American Occupational Therapy Association. (2007a). Accreditation standards for a doctoral-degree-level educational program for the occupational therapist. *American Journal of Occupational Therapy, 61,* 641–651.

American Occupational Therapy Association. (2007b). Accreditation standards for a master's-degree-level educational program for the occupational therapist. *American Journal of Occupational Therapy, 61,* 652–661.

American Occupational Therapy Association. (2007c). Accreditation standards for an educational program for the occupational therapy assistant. *American Journal of Occupational Therapy, 61,* 662–671.

American Occupational Therapy Association. (2007d). Specialized knowledge and skills in feeding, eating, and swallowing for occupational therapy practice. *American Journal of Occupational Therapy, 61,* 686–700.

American Occupational Therapy Association. (2008a). Guidelines for documentation of occupational therapy. *American Journal of Occupational Therapy, 62,* 684–690.

American Occupational Therapy Association. (2008b). Occupational therapy practice framework: Domain and process (2nd ed.). *American Journal of Occupational Therapy, 62,* 625–683.

Anderson, C. S., Hackett, M. L., & House, A. O. (2004). Interventions for preventing depression after stroke. *Cochrane Database of Systematic Reviews,* Issue No. 2, Art. No. CD003689.

Arnadottir, G. (1990). *The brain and behavior: Assessing cortical dysfunction through activities of daily living.* St. Louis, MO: Mosby.

Asanuma, H., & Pavlides, C. (1997). Neurobiological basis of motor learning in mammals. *Neuroreport, 8,* 1–6.

Ashworth, B. (1964). Preliminary trial of carisprodal in multiple sclerosis. *Practitioner, 192,* 540–542.

Avery-Smith, W., & Dellarosa, D. M. (1994). Approaches to treating dysphagia in patients with brain injury. *American Journal of Occupational Therapy, 48,* 235–239.

Bagg, S. D. & Forrest, W. F. (1988). A biomechanical analysis of scapular rotation during arm abduction in the scapular plane. *American Journal of Physical Medicine and Rehabilitation, 67,* 238–245.

Barreca, S., Gowland, C. K., Stratford, P., Huijbregts, M., Griffiths, J., Torresin, W., et al. (2004). Development of the Chedoke Arm and Hand Activity Inventory: Theoretical constructs, item generation, and selection. *Topics in Stroke Rehabilitation, 4,* 31–42.

Barreca, S., Wolf, S. L., Fasoli, S., & Bohannon, R. (2003). Treatment interventions for the paretic upper limb of stroke survivors: A critical review. *Neurorehabilitation and Neural Repair, 17,* 220–226.

Baum, C. M. & Edwards. D. (2008). *Activity Card Sort* (2nd ed.). Bethesda, MD: AOTA Press.

Berg, K., Wood-Dauphinee, S., Williams, J., & Gayton, D. (1989). Measuring balance in the elderly: Preliminary development of an instrument. *Physiotherapy Canada, 41,* 304–311.

Biernaskie, J., & Corbett, D. (2001). Enriched rehabilitative training promotes improved forelimb motor function and enhanced dendritic growth after focal ischemic injury. *Journal of Neuroscience, 21,* 5272–5280.

Binkofski, F., Seitz, R. J., Arnold, S., Classen, J., Benecke, R., & Freund, H. J. (1996). Thalamic metabolism and corticospinal tract integrity determine motor recovery in stroke. *Annals of Neurology, 39,* 460–470.

Bobath, B. (1978). *Adult hemiplegia: Evaluation and treatment.* London: Heinemann.

Bode, R. K., Heinemann, A. W., Semik, P., & Mallinson, T. (2004). Relative importance of rehabilitation therapy characteristics on functional outcomes for persons with stroke. *Stroke, 35,* 2537–2542.

Bohannan, R. W., & Andrews, A. W. (1990). Shoulder subluxation and pain in stroke patients. *American Journal of Occupational Therapy, 44,* 507–509.

Bourne, D. A., Choo, A. M., Regan, W. D., MacIntyre, D. L., & Oxland, T. R. (2007). Three-dimensional rotation of the scapula during functional movements: An in vivo study in healthy volunteers. *Journal of Shoulder and Elbow Surgery, 16,* 150–162.

Bowen, A., Lincoln, N. B., & Dewey, M. (2002). Cognitive rehabilitation for spatial neglect following stroke. *Cochrane Database of Systematic Reviews,* Issue No. 2, Art. No. CD003586.

Brogardh, C., & Sjölund, B. H. (2006). Constraint-induced movement therapy in patients with stroke: A pilot study on effects of small group training and of extended mitt use. *Clinical Rehabilitation, 20,* 218–227.

Brown, A. W., Bjelke, B., & Fuxe, K. (2004). Motor response to amphetamine treatment, task-specific training, and limited motor experience in a postacute animal stroke model. *Experimental Neurology, 190*, 102–108.

Buschbacher, R. M. (1996). Deconditioning, conditioning, and the benefits of exercise. In R. L. Braddom (Ed.), *Physical medicine and rehabilitation* (pp. 687–708). Philadelphia: W. B. Saunders.

Butefisch, C. M. (2004). Plasticity in the human cerebral cortex: Lessons from the normal brain and from stroke. *Neuroscientist, 10*, 163–173.

Calautti, C., & Baron, J. C. (2003). Functional neuroimaging studies of motor recovery after stroke in adults: A review. *Stroke, 34*, 1553–1556.

Carr, J. H., & Shepherd, R. B. (1998). *Neurological rehabilitation: Optimizing motor performance.* Oxford: Butterworth-Heinemann.

Carr, J. H., & Shepherd, R. B. (2003). *Stroke rehabilitation: Guidelines for exercise and training to optimize motor skill.* Boston: Butterworth-Heinemann.

Carr, J. H., Shepherd, R. B., Nordholm, L., & Lynne, D. (1985). Investigation of a new motor assessment scale for stroke patients. *Physical Therapy, 65*, 175–180.

Center for Functional Assessment Research at the State University of New York at Buffalo. (1993). *Functional Independence Measure* (4th ed.). Buffalo, NY: Data Management Service of the Uniform Data System for Medical Rehabilitation.

Choi-Kwon, S., Han, S. W., Kwon, S. U., & Kim, J. S. (2005). Poststroke fatigue: Characteristics and related factors. *Cerebrovascular Disease, 19*, 84–90.

Clarke, P., Marshall, V., Black, S. E., & Colantonio, A. (2002). Well-being after stroke in Canadian seniors: Findings from the Canadian study of health and aging. *Stroke, 33*, 1016–1021.

Clemson, L., Cumming, R. G., Kendig, H., Swann, M., Heard, R., & Taylor, K. (2004). The effectiveness of a community-based program for reducing the incidence of falls in the elderly: A randomized trial. *Journal of the American Geriatrics Society, 52*, 1487–1494.

Colarusso, R. P., & Hammill, D. D. (2003). *Motor-Free Visual Perception Test (MVPT–3*, 3rd ed.). Novato, CA: Academic Therapy Publications.

Corr, S., & Bayer, A. (1995). Occupational therapy for stroke patients after hospital discharge—A randomized controlled trial. *Clinical Rehabilitation, 9*, 291–296.

Cramer, S. C., Nelles, G., Benson, R. R., Kaplan, J. D., Parker, R. A., Kwong, K. K., et al. (1997). A functional MRI study of subjects recovered from hemiparetic stroke. *Stroke, 28*, 2518–2527.

Dahlqvist, P., Ronnback, A., Bergstrom, S. A., Soderstrom, I., & Olsson, T. (2004). Environmental enrichment reverses learning impairment in the Morris water maze after focal cerebral ischemia in rats. *European Journal of Neuroscience, 19*, 2288–2298.

Dancause, N. (2006). Neurophysiological and anatomical plasticity in the adult sensorimotor cortex. *Reviews in the Neurosciences, 17*, 561–580.

Dean, C. M., & Shepherd, R. B. (1997). Task-related training improves performance of seated reaching tasks after stroke: A randomized controlled trial. *Stroke, 28*, 722–728.

Diller, L., Ben-Yishay, Y., Gertsman, L. J., Goodin, R., Gordon, W., & Weinberg, J. (1974). Studies in scanning behavior in hemiplegia. *Rehabilitation Monograph No. 50, Studies in cognition and rehabilitation in hemiplegia.* New York: New York University Medical Center, Institute of Rehabilitation Medicine.

Dirette, D., & Hinojosa, J. (1994). Effects of continuous passive motion on the edematous hands of two persons with flaccid hemiplegia. *American Journal of Occupational Therapy, 48*, 403–409.

Dolecheck, J. R., & Schkade, J. K. (1999). The extent dynamic standing endurance is effected when CVA subjects perform personally meaningful activities rather than nonmeaningful tasks. *Occupational Therapy Journal of Research, 19*, 40–54.

Donkervoort M., Dekker J., Stehmann-Saris, F. C., & Deelman, B. G. (2001). Effect of strategy training in left hemisphere stroke patients with apraxia: A randomized clinical trial. *Neuropsychological Rehabilitation, 11*, 549–566.

Drummond, A. E. R., & Walker, M. F. (1995). A randomized controlled trial of leisure rehabilitation after stroke. *Clinical Rehabilitation, 9*, 283–290.

Drummond, A. E. R., & Walker, M. F. (1996). Generalisation of the effects of leisure rehabilitation for stroke patients. *British Journal of Occupational Therapy, 59*, 330–334.

Duncan, P. W., Bode, R. K., Min Lai, S., & Perera, S. (2003). Glycine antagonist in neuroprotection Americans investigators. *Archives of Physical Medicine and Rehabilitation, 84*, 950–963.

Duncan, P. W., Wallace, D., Lai, S. M., Johnson, D., Embretson, S., & Laster, L. J. (1999). The Stroke Impact Scale Version 2.0. Evaluation of reliability, validity, and sensitivity to change. *Stroke, 30*, 2131–2140.

Duncan, P. W., Weiner, D. K., Chandler, J., & Studenski, S. (1990). Functional reach: A new clinical measure of balance. *Journal of Gerontology: Medical Sciences, 45*, M192–M197.

Duncan, P. W., Zorowitz, R., Bates, B., Choi, J. Y., Glasberg, J. J., Graham, G. D., et al. (2005). AHA/ASA–endorsed practice guidelines: Management of adult stroke rehabilitation care. *Stroke, 36*, 100–143.

Dursun, E., Dursun, N., Ural, C. E., & Cakci, A. (2000). Glenohumeral joint subluxation and reflex sympathetic dystrophy in hemiplegic patients. *Archives of Physical Medicine and Rehabilitation, 81*, 944–946.

Faghri, P. D., Rodgers, M. M., Glaser, R. M., Bors, J. G., Ho, C., & Akuthota, P. (1994). The effects of functional electrical stimulation on shoulder subluxation, arm function, recovery, and shoulder pain in hemiplegic stroke patients. *Archives of Physical Medicine and Rehabilitation, 75*, 73–79.

Fasoli, S. E., Krebs, H. I., Stein, J., Frontera, W. R., & Hogan, N. (2003). Effects of robotic therapy on motor impairment and recovery in chronic stroke. *Archives of Physical Medicine and Rehabilitation, 84*, 477–482.

Fasoli, S. E., Trombly, C. A., Tickle-Degnen, L., & Verfaellie, M. H. (2002). Effect of instructions on functional reach in persons with and without cerebrovascular accident. *American Journal of Occupational Therapy, 56*, 380–390.

Fischer, A. G. (1995). *Assessment of Motor and Process Skills.* Fort Collins, CO: Three Star Press.

Fischer, S., Gauggel, S., & Trexler, L. E. (2004). Awareness of activity limitations, goal setting, and rehabilitation outcome in patients with brain injuries. *Brain Injury, 18*, 547–562.

Flinn, N. A., Schamburg, S., Fetrow, J. M., & Flanigan, J. (2005). The effect of constraint-induced movement treatment on occupational performance and satisfaction in stroke survivors. *OTJR: Occupation, Participation and Health, 25*, 119–127.

Foltys, H., Krings, T., Meister, I. G., Sparing, R., Boroojerdi, B., Thron, A., et al. (2003). Motor representation in patients rapidly recovering after stroke: A functional magnetic resonance imaging and transcranial magnetic stimulation study. *Clinical Neurophysiology, 114*, 2404–2415.

Fong, K. N., Chan, C. C., & Au, D. K. (2001). Relationship of motor and cognitive abilities to functional performance in stroke rehabilitation. *Brain Injury, 15*, 443–453.

Freedman, L., & Munro, R. (1966). Abduction of the arm in the scapular plane: Scapular and glenohumeral movements. *Journal of Bone and Joint Surgery, 48A*, 1503–1510.

French, B., Thomas, L. H., Leathley, M. J., Sutton, C. J., McAdam, J., Forster, A., et al. (2007). Repetitive task training for improving functional ability after stroke. *Cochrane Database of Systematic Reviews*, Issue No. 4, Art. No. CD006073.

Friel, K. M., Heddings, A. A., & Nudo, R. J. (2000). Effects of postlesion experience on behavioral recovery and neurophysiologic reorganization after cortical injury in primates. *Neurorehabilitation and Neural Repair, 14*, 187–198.

Fritz, S. L., Light, K. E., Clifford, S. N., Patterson, T. S., Behrman, A. L., & Davis, S. B. (2006). Descriptive characteristics as potential predictors of outcomes following constraint-induced movement therapy for people after stroke. *Physical Therapy, 86*, 825–832.

Fugl-Meyer, A., Jaasko, L., Leyman, I., Olsson, S., & Steglind, S. (1975). The post-stroke hemiplegic patient: 1. A method for evaluation of physical performance. *Scandinavian Journal of Rehabilitation Medicine, 7*, 13–31.

Geurts, A. C., Visschers, B. A., van Limbeek, J., & Ribbers, G. M. (2000). Systematic review of aetiology and treatment of post-stroke hand oedema and shoulder-hand syndrome. *Scandinavian Journal of Rehabilitation Medicine, 32*, 4–10.

Geusgens, C. A. V., van Heugten, C. M., Cooijmans, J. P. J., Jolles, J., & van den Heuvel, W. J. A. (2006). Transfer effects of a cognitive strategy training for stroke patients with apraxia. *Journal of Clinical and Experimental Neuropsychology, 29*, 831–841.

Geusgens, C. A. V., Winkens, L., van Heugten, C. M., Jolles, J., & van den Heuvel, W. J. A. (2007). Occurrence and measurement of transfer in cognitive rehabilitation: A critical review. *Journal of Rehabilitation Medicine, 39*, 425–439.

Gibson, J. W., & Schkade, J. K. (1997). Occupational adaptation intervention with patients with cerebrovascular accident: A clinical study. *American Journal of Occupational Therapy, 51*, 523–529.

Gilbertson, L., Langhorne, P., Walker, A., Allen, A., & Murray, G. D. (2000). Domiciliary occupational therapy for patients with stroke discharged from hospital: Randomised controlled trial. *British Medical Journal, 320*, 603–606.

Gillen, G., & Burkhardt, A. (2004). *Stroke rehabilitation: A function-based approach* (2nd ed.). St. Louis, MO: Mosby.

Giuffrida, C. G., Shea, J. B., & Fairbrother, J. T. (2002). Differential transfer benefits of increased practice for constant, blocked, and serial practice schedules. *Journal of Motor Behavior, 34*, 353–365.

Gladman, J. R. R., Lincoln, N. B., & Adams, S. A. (1993). Use of the extended ADL scale with stroke patients. *Age and Ageing, 22*, 419–424.

Goldenberg, G., Hentze, S., & Hermsdörfer, J. (2004). The effect of tactile feedback on pantomime of tool use in apraxia. *Neurology, 63*, 1863–1867.

Goodglass, H., & Kaplan, E. (1972). *The assessment of aphasia and related disorders.* Philadelphia: Lea & Febiger.

Greenberg, S., & Fowler, R. S., Jr. (1980). Kinesthetic biofeedback: A treatment modality for elbow range of motion in hemiplegia. *American Journal of Occupational Therapy, 34*, 738–743.

Gresham, G. E., Duncan, P. W., Stason, W. B., Adams, H. P., Adelman, A. M., Alexander, D. N., et al. (1995). *Post-stroke rehabilitation.* Clinical Practice Guideline No. 16 (AHCPR Pub. No. 95-0062). Rockville, MD: U.S. Department of Health and Human Services, Public Health Service, Agency for Health Care Policy and Research.

Hall, K. G., & Magill, R. A. (1995). Variability of practice and contextual interference in motor skill learning. *Journal of Motor Behavior, 27*, 299–309.

Hanger, H. C., Whitewood, P., Brown, G., Ball, M. C., Harper, J., Cox, R., et al. (2000). A randomized controlled trial of strapping to prevent post-stroke shoulder pain. *Clinical Rehabilitation, 14*, 370–380.

Hayes, R. L., & McGrath, J. J. (1998). Evidence-based practice: The Cochrane collaboration and occupational therapy. *La Revue Canadienne D'Ergotherapie, 65*, 141–151.

Heilman, K. M., & Valenstein, E. (1979). Mechanisms underlying hemispatial neglect. *Annals of Neurology, 5,* 166–170.

Higgins, J. P. T., & Green, S. (Eds.). (2005). *Cochrane handbook for systematic reviews of interventions 4.2.5.* Retrieved May 31, 2006, from http://www.cochrane.org/resources/handbook/hbook.htm

Holm, M. B., Rogers, J. C., & Stone, R. G. (2003). Person–task–environment interventions: A decision-making guide. In E. B. Crepeau, E. S. Cohn, & B. A. Boyt Schell (Eds.), *Willard and Spackman's occupational therapy* (10th ed., pp. 460–490). Philadelphia: Lippincott, Williams & Wilkins.

Howle, J. M. (2002). *Neuro-developmental treatment approach: Theoretical foundations and principles of clinical practice.* Laguna Beach, CA: North American Neurodevelopmental Treatment Association.

Hsieh, C. L., Nelson, D. L., Smith, D. A., & Peterson, C. Q. (1996). A comparison of performance in added-purpose occupations and rote exercise for dynamic standing balance in persons with hemiplegia. *American Journal of Occupational Therapy, 50,* 10–16.

Humm, J. L., Kozlowski, D. A., James, D. C., Gotts, J. E., & Schallert, T. (1998). Use-dependent exacerbation of brain damage occurs during an early postlesion vulnerable period. *Brain Research, 783,* 286–292.

Ingles, J. L., Eskes, G. A., & Phillips, S. J. (1999). Fatigue after stroke. *Archives of Physical Medicine and Rehabilitation, 80,* 173–178.

Inman, V. T., Saunders, M., & Abbott, L. C. (1944). Observations on the function of the shoulder joint. *Journal of Bone and Joint Surgery, 26A,* 1–32.

Johansen-Berg, H., Dawes, H., Guy, C., Smith, S. M., Wade, D. T., & Matthews, P. M. (2002). Correlation between motor improvements and altered ƒMRI activity after rehabilitative therapy. *Brain, 135,* 2731–2742.

Johansson, B. B. (1996). Functional outcome in rats transferred to an enriched environment 15 days after focal brain ischemia. *Stroke, 27,* 324–326.

Johansson, B. B. (2003). Environmental influence on recovery after brain lesions: Experimental and clinical data. *Journal of Rehabilitation Medicine, 41*(Suppl.), 11–16.

Jones, T. A., Chu, C. J., Grande, L. A., & Gregory, A. D. (1999). Motor skills training enhances lesion-induced structural plasticity in the motor cortex of adult rats. *Journal of Neuroscience, 19,* 10153–10163.

Jongbloed, L., & Morgan, D. (1991). An investigation of involvement in leisure activities after a stroke. *American Journal of Occupational Therapy, 45,* 420–427.

Jongbloed, L., Stacey, S., & Brighton, C. (1989). Stroke rehabilitation: Sensorimotor integrative treatment versus functional treatment. *American Journal of Occupational Therapy, 43,* 391–397.

Jonsson, A. C., Lindgren, I., Hallstrom, B., Norrving, B., & Lindgren, A. (2005). Determinants of quality of life in stroke survivors and their informal caregivers. *Stroke, 36,* 803–808.

Jorgensen, H. S., Nakayama, H., Raaschou, H. O., Vive-Larsen, J., Stoier, M., & Olsen, T. S. (1995). Outcome and time course of recovery in stroke. Part I: Outcome. The Copenhagen Stroke Study. *Archives of Physical Medicine and Rehabilitation, 76,* 399–405.

Katz, N. (2005). *Cognition and occupation across the life span* (2nd ed.). Bethesda, MD: AOTA Press.

Katz, N., Itzkovich, M., Averbuch, S., & Elazar, B. (1989). Loewenstein Occupational Therapy Cognitive Assessment (LOTCA) Battery for brain-injured patients: Reliability and validity. *American Journal of Occupational Therapy, 43,* 184–192.

Kautzmann, L. N. (1984). Identifying leisure interests: A self-assessment approach for adults with arthritis. *Occupational Therapy in Health Care, 1,* 45–52.

Kennedy, L. E., & Bhambhani, Y. N. (1991). The Baltimore Therapeutic Equipment Work Simulator: Reliability and validity at three work intensities. *Archives of Physical Medicine and Rehabilitation, 72*, 511–516.

Kopp, B., Kunkel, A., Flor, H., Platz, T., Rose, U., Mauritz, K. H., et al. (1997). The Arm Motor Ability Test: Reliability, validity, and sensitivity to change of an instrument for assessing disabilities in activities of daily living. *Archives of Physical Medicine and Rehabilitation, 78*, 615–620.

Kumar, R., Metter, E. J., Mehta, A. J., & Chew, T. (1990). Shoulder pain in hemiplegia: The role of exercise. *American Journal of Physical Medicine and Rehabilitation, 69*, 205–208.

Kunkel, A., Kopp, B., Muller, G., Villringer, K., Villringer, A., Taub, E., et al. (1999). Constraint-induced movement therapy for motor recovery in chronic stroke patients. *Archives of Physical Medicine and Rehabilitation, 80*, 624–628.

Langhorne, P., & Pollock, A. (2002). What are the components of effective stroke unit care? *Age and Ageing, 31*, 365–371.

Lannin, N. A., & Herbert, R. D. (2003). Is hand splinting effective for adults following stroke? A systematic review and methodologic critique of published research. *Clinical Rehabilitation, 17*, 807–816.

Law, M., Baptiste, S., Carswell, A., McColl, M., Polatajko, H., & Pollock, N. (1998). *Canadian Occupational Performance Measure manual* (3rd ed.). Ottawa: CAOT Publications.

Law, M., & Baum, C. (1998). Evidenced-based occupational therapy. *Canadian Journal of Occupational Therapy, 65*, 131–135.

Leasure, J. L., & Schallert, T. (2004). Consequences of forced disuse of the impaired forelimb after unilateral cortical injury. *Behavioral Brain Research, 150*, 83–91.

Legg, L. A., Drummond, A. E., & Langhorne, P. (2006). Occupational therapy for patients with problems in activities of daily living after stroke. *Cochrane Database of Systematic Reviews*, Issue No. 4, Art. No. CD003585.

Lenze, E. J., Munin, M. C., Quear, T., Dew, M. A., Rogers, J. C., Begley, A. E., et al. (2004). Significance of poor patient participation in physical and occupational therapy for functional outcome and length of stay. *Archives of Physical Medicine and Rehabilitation, 85*, 1599–1601.

Levine, P., & Page, S. J. (2004). Modified constraint-induced therapy: A promising restorative outpatient therapy. *Topics in Stroke Rehabilitation, 11*, 1–10.

Liepert, J. (2006). Motor cortex excitability in stroke before and after constraint-induced movement therapy. *Cognitive and Behavioral Neurology, 19*, 41–47.

Liepert, J., Bauder, H., Wolfgang, H. R., Miltner, W. H., Taub, E., & Weiller, C. (2000). Treatment-induced cortical reorganization after stroke in humans. *Stroke, 31*, 1210–1216.

Liepert, J., Hamzei, F., & Weiller, C. (2004). Lesion-induced and training-induced brain reorganization. *Restorative Neurology and Neuroscience, 22*, 269–277.

Lin, K.-C., Cermak, S. A., Kinsbourne, M., & Trombly, C. A. (1996). Effects of left-sided movements on line bisection in unilateral neglect. *Journal of the International Neuropsychological Society, 2*, 404–411.

Lin, K.-C., Wu, C. Y., Tickle-Degnen, L., & Coster, W. (1997). Enhancing occupational performance through occupationally embedded exercise: A meta-analytic review. *Occupational Therapy Journal of Research, 17*, 25–47.

Lin, K.-C., Wu, C.-Y., Wei, T. H., Lee, C. Y., & Liu, J. S. (2007). Effects of modified constraint-induced movement therapy on reach-to-grasp movements and functional performance after chronic stroke: A randomized controlled study. *Clinical Rehabilitation, 21,* 1075–1086.

Lincoln, N. B., Drummond, A. E., & Berman, P. (1997). Perceptual impairment and its impact on rehabilitation outcomes. *Disability and Rehabilitation, 19,* 231–234.

Linden, A., Boschian, K., Eker, C., Schalen, W., & Nordstrom, C. H. (2005). Assessment of motor and process skills reflects brain-injured patients' ability to resume independent living better than neuropsychological tests. *Acta Neurologica Scandinavia, 111,* 48–53.

Logan, P. A., Ahern, J., Gladman, J. R. F., & Lincoln, N. G. (1997). A randomized controlled trial of enhanced social service occupational therapy for stroke patients. *Clinical Rehabilitation, 11,* 107–113.

Logan, P. A., Gladman, J. R. F., Avery, A., Walker, M. F., Dyas, J., & Groom, L. (2004). Randomised controlled trial of an occupational therapy intervention to increase outdoor mobility after stroke. *British Medical Journal, 329,* 1372–1375.

Luke, C., Dodd, K. J., & Brock, K. (2004). Outcomes of the Bobath concept on upper limb recovery following stroke. *Clinical Rehabilitation, 18,* 888–898.

Lum, P. S., Burgar, C. G., Shor, P. C., Majmundar, M., & Van der Loos, M. (2002). Robot-assisted movement training compared with conventional therapy techniques for the rehabilitation of upper-limb motor function after stroke. *Archives of Physical Medicine and Rehabilitation, 83,* 952–959.

Ma, H.-I., & Trombly, C. A. (2002). A synthesis of the effects of occupational therapy for persons with stroke, part II: Remediation. *American Journal of Occupational Therapy, 56,* 260–274.

Ma, H.-I., Trombly, C. A., & Robinson-Podolski, C. (1999). The effect of context on skill acquisition and transfer. *American Journal of Occupational Therapy, 53,* 138–144.

Majid, M. J., Lincoln, N. B., & Weyman, N. (2000). Cognitive rehabilitation for memory deficits following stroke. *Cochrane Database of Systematic Reviews,* Issue No. 2, Art. No. CD002293.

Malec, J., Zweber, B., & DePompolo, R. (1990). The Rivermead Behavioural Memory Test, laboratory neurocognitive measures, and everyday functioning. *Journal of Head Trauma Rehabilitation, 5,* 60–68.

Mark, V. W., & Taub, E. (2004). Constraint-induced movement therapy for chronic stroke hemiparesis and other disabilities. *Restorative Neurology and Neuroscience, 22,* 317–336.

Mathias, S., Nayak, U., & Issacs, B. (1986). Balance in elderly patients: The "Get Up and Go" test. *Archives of Physical Medicine and Rehabilitation, 67,* 387–389.

Mathiowetz, V., Bolding, D. J., & Trombly, C. A. (1983). Immediate effects of positioning devices on the normal and spastic hand measured by electromyography. *American Journal of Occupational Therapy, 37,* 247–254.

Mayo, N. E., Wood-Dauphinee, S., Cote, R., Durcan, L., & Carlton, J. (2002). Activity, participation, and quality of life 6 months poststroke. *Archives of Physical Medicine and Rehabilitation, 83,* 1035–1042.

Morris, D. M., Uswatte, G., Crago, J. E., Cook, E. W., & Taub, E. (2001). The reliability of the Wolf Motor Function Test for assessing upper extremity function after stroke. *Archives of Physical Medicine and Rehabilitation, 82,* 750–755.

Morris, S. L., Dodd, K. J., & Morris, M. E. (2004). Outcomes of progressive resistance strength training following stroke: A systematic review. *Clinical Rehabilitation, 18,* 27–39.

Mosey, A. C. (1996). *Applied scientific inquiry in the health professions: An epistemological orientation* (2nd ed.). Bethesda, MD: American Occupational Therapy Association.

Moyers, P. A., & Dale, L. M. (2007). *The guide to occupational therapy practice* (2nd ed.). Bethesda, MD: AOTA Press.

Mudie, M. H., Winzeler-Mercay, U., Radwan, S., & Lee, L. (2002). Training symmetry of weight distribution after stroke: A randomized controlled pilot study comparing task-related reach, Bobath and feedback training approaches. *Clinical Rehabilitation, 16,* 582–592.

Muraki, T., Kujime, K., Su, M., Kaneko, T., & Ueba, Y. (1990). Effect of one hand sanding on cardiometabolic and ventilatory functions in the hemiplegic elderly: A preliminary investigation. *Physical and Occupational Therapy in Geriatrics, 9,* 37–48.

Nelson, D. L., Konosky, K., Fleharty, K., Webb, R., Newer, K., Hazboun, V. P., et al. (1996). The effects of an occupationally embedded exercise on bilaterally assisted supination in persons with hemiplegia. *American Journal of Occupational Therapy, 50,* 639–646.

New Zealand Guidelines Group. (2003). *Life after stroke: New Zealand guideline for management of stroke.* Wellington, New Zealand: Author. (Available through National Guideline Clearinghouse, www.guideline.gov.)

Norbeck, J. S., Lindsey, A. M., & Carrieri, V. L. (1981). The development of an instrument to measure social support. *Nursing Research, 32,* 4–9.

Nudo, R. J., (2003). Functional and structural plasticity in motor cortex: Implications for stroke recovery. *Physical Medicine and Physical Rehabilitation Clinics of North America. 14,* S57–S76.

Nudo, R. J., Milliken, G. W., Jenkins, W. M., & Merzenich, M. M. (1996). Use-dependent alterations of movement representations in primary motor cortex of adult squirrel monkeys. *Journal of Neuroscience, 16,* 785–807.

Oakley, F., Kielhofner, G., Barris, R., & Reichler, R. K. (1986). The Role Checklist: Development and empirical assessment of reliability. *Occupational Therapy Journal of Research, 6,* 157–169.

Ostendorf, C. G., & Wolf, S. L. (1981). Effect of forced use of the upper extremity of a hemiplegic patient on changes in function. *Physical Therapy, 61,* 1022–1028.

Ottawa Panel. (2006). Evidence-based clinical practice guidelines for poststroke rehabilitation [Special issue]. *Topics in Stroke Rehabilitation, 13,* 1–269.

Outpatient Service Trialists. (2004). Rehabilitation therapy services for stroke patients living at home: Systematic review of randomized trials. *Lancet, 363,* 352–356.

Paci, M. (2003). Physiotherapy based on the Bobath concept for adults with poststroke hemiplegia: A review of effectiveness studies. *Journal of Rehabilitation Medicine, 35,* 2–7.

Paci, M., Nannetti, L., Taiti, P., Baccini, M., & Rinaldi, L. (2007). Shoulder subluxation after stroke: Relationships with pain and motor recovery. *Physiotherapy Research International, 12,* 95–104.

Page, S. J., & Levine, P. (2006). Back from the brink: Electromyography-triggered stimulation combined with modified constraint-induced movement therapy in chronic stroke. *Archives of Physical Medicine and Rehabilitation, 87,* 27–31.

Page, S. J., Levine, P., Leonard, A., Szaflarski, J. P., & Kissela, B. M. (2008). Modified constraint-induced therapy in chronic stroke: Results of a single-blinded randomized controlled trial. *Physical Therapy, 88,* 1–8.

Page, S. J., Sisto, S., Levine, P., & McGrath, R. E. (2004). Efficacy of modified constraint-induced movement therapy in chronic stroke: A single-blinded randomized controlled trial. *Archives of Physical Medicine and Rehabilitation, 85,* 14–18.

Parham, L. D., & Fazio, L. S. (Eds.). (1997). *Play in occupational therapy for children.* St. Louis, MO: Mosby.

Parker, C. J., Gladman, J. R., Drummond, A. E., Dewey, M. E., Lincoln, N. B., Barer, D., et al. (2001). A multicentre randomized controlled trial of leisure therapy and conventional occupational therapy after stroke. TOTAL Study Group. Trial of occupational therapy and leisure. *Clinical Rehabilitation, 15,* 42–52.

Patten, C., Lexell, J., & Brown, H. E. (2004). Weakness and strength training in persons with poststroke hemiplegia: Rationale, method, and efficacy. *Journal of Rehabilitation Research and Development, 41,* 293–312.

Pellecchia, G. L. (2004). Figure-of-eight method of measuring hand size: Reliability and concurrent validity. *Journal of Hand Therapy, 16,* 300–304.

Plautz, E. J., Milliken, G. W., & Nudo, R. J. (2000). Effects of repetitive motor training on movement representations in adult squirrel monkeys: Role of use versus learning. *Neurobiology of Learning and Memory, 74,* 27–55.

Pollock, A., Baer, G., Pomeroy, V., & Langhorne, P. (2007). Physiotherapy treatment approaches for the recovery of postural control and lower limb function following stroke. *Cochrane Database of Systematic Reviews,* Issue No. 1, Art. No. CD001920.

Pomeroy, V. M., King, L., Pollock, A., Baily-Hallam, A., & Langhorne, P. (2006). Electrostimulation for promoting recovery of movement or functional ability after stroke. *Cochrane Database of Systematic Reviews,* Issue No. 2, Art. No. CD003241.

Poole, J. L. (1998). Effect of apraxia on the ability to learn one-handed shoe tying. *Occupational Therapy Journal of Research, 18,* 99–104.

Poole, J. L., Whitney, S. L., Hangeland, N., & Baker, C. (1990). The effectiveness of inflatable pressure splints on motor function in stroke patients. *Occupational Therapy Journal of Research, 10,* 360–366.

Prange, G. B., Jannink, M. J. A., Groothuis-Oudshoorn, C. G. M., Hermens, H. J., & Ijzerman, M. J. (2006). Systematic review of the effect of robot-aided therapy on recovery of the hemiparetic arm after stroke. *Journal of Rehabilitation Research and Development, 43,* 171–184.

Price, C. I. M., & Pandyan, A. D. (2000). Electrical stimulation for preventing and treating post-stroke shoulder pain. *Database of Systematic Reviews,* Issue No. 4, Art. No. CD001698.

Radomski, M. V., & Trombly Latham, C. A. (2008). *Occupational therapy for physical dysfunction* (6th ed.). Philadelphia: Lippincott Williams & Wilkins.

Ro, T., Noser, E., Boake, C., Johnson, R. Gaber, M., Speroni, A., et al. (2006). Functional reorganization and recovery after constraint-induced movement therapy in subacute stroke: Case reports. *Neurocase, 12,* 50–60.

Robertson, I. H., Ward, T., Ridgeway, V., & Nimmo-Smith, I. 1996. The structure of normal human attention: The Test of Everyday Attention. *Journal of the International Neuropsychological Society, 2,* 525–534.

Rogers, J., & Holm, M. (1994). Assessment of self-care. In B. R. Bonder & M. B. Wagner (Eds.), *Functional performance in older adults* (pp. 181–202). Philadelphia: F. A. Davis.

Rossini, P. M., Altamura, C., Ferreri, F., Melgari, J. M., Tecchio, F., Tombini, M., et al. (2007). Neuroimaging experimental studies on brain plasticity in recovery from stroke. *Europa Medicophysiology, 43,* 241–254.

Roth, E. J., Heinemann, A. W., Lovell, L. L., Harvey, R. L., McGuire, J. R., & Diaz, S. (1998). Impairment and disability: Their relation during stroke rehabilitation. *Archives of Physical Medicine and Rehabilitation, 79,* 329–335.

Sackett, D. L., Rosenberg, W. M., Muir Gray, J. A., Haynes, R. B., & Richardson, W. S. (1996). Evidence-based medicine: What it is and what it isn't. *British Medical Journal, 312*, 71–72.

Sadato, N., Pascual-Leone, A., Grafman, J., Deiber, M. P., Ibanez, V., & Hallett, M. (1998). Neural networks for Braille reading by the blind. *Brain, 121*, 1213–1229.

Saito, D. N., Okada, T., Honda, M., Yonekura, Y., & Sadato, N. (2006). Practice makes perfect: The neural substrates of tactile discrimination by Mah-Jong experts include the primary visual cortex. *BMC Neuroscience, 7*, 79–89.

Schaechter, J. D. (2004). Motor rehabilitation and brain plasticity after hemiparetic stroke. *Progress in Neurobiology, 73*, 61–72.

Schmidt, R. A., & Lee, T. D. (2005). *Motor control and learning: A behavioral emphasis* (4th ed.). Champaign, IL: Human Kinetics.

Scottish Intercollegiate Guidelines Network. (2002). *Management of patients with stroke: Rehabilitation, prevention and management of complications, and discharge planning. A national clinical guideline.* Edinburgh: Author.

Shumway-Cook, A., & Woollacott, M. H. (2006). *Motor control: Translating research into clinical practice.* Philadelphia: Lippincott Williams & Wilkins.

Smedley, R. R., Fiorino, A. J., Soucar, E., Reynolds, D., Smedley, W. P., & Aronica, M. J. (1986). Slot machines: Their use in rehabilitation after stroke. *Archives of Physical Medicine and Rehabilitation, 67*, 546–549.

Smithard, D. G., O'Neill, P. A., England, R. E., Park, C. L., Wyatt, R., Martin, D. F., et al. (1997). The natural history of dysphagia following a stroke. *Dysphagia, 13*, 230–231.

Snels, I. A., Dekker, J. H., van der Lee, J. H., Lankhorst, G. J., Beckerman, H., & Bouter, L. M. (2002). Treating patients with hemiplegic shoulder pain. *American Journal of Physical Medicine and Rehabilitation, 81*, 150–160.

Söderback, I. (1988). The effectiveness of training intellectual functions in adults with acquired brain damage: An evaluation of occupational therapy methods. *Scandinavian Journal of Rehabilitation Medicine, 20*, 47–56.

Stav, W. B., Hunt, L. A., & Arbesman, M. (2006). *Occupational therapy practice guidelines for driving and community mobility for older adults.* Bethesda, MD: American Occupational Therapy Association.

Sterr, A., Elbert, T., Berthold, I., Kolbel, S., Rockstroh, B., & Taub, E. (2002). Longer versus shorter daily constraint-induced movement therapy of chronic hemiparesis: An exploratory study. *Archives of Physical Medicine and Rehabilitation, 83*, 1374–1377.

Steultjens, E. M. J., Dekker, J., Bouter, L. M., van de Nes, J. C. M., Cup, E. H. D., & van den Ende, C. H. M. (2003). Occupational therapy for stroke patients: A systematic review. *Stroke, 34*, 676–687.

Stokdijk, M., Eilers, P. H., Nagels, J., & Rozing, P. M. (2003). External rotation in the glenohumeral joint during elevation of the arm. *Clinical Biomechanics, 18*, 296–302.

Stroke Canada Optimization of Rehabilitation through Evidence (SCORE). (2007). *SCORE evidence-based recommendations for the upper and lower extremities and risk assessment post-stroke, 2007.* Toronto: Author.

Szaflarski, J. P., Page, S. P., Kissela, B. M., Lee, J.-H., Levine, P., & Strakowski, S. M. (2006). Cortical reorganization following modified constraint-induced movement therapy: A study of 4 patients with chronic stroke. *Archives of Physical Medicine and Rehabilitation, 87*, 1052–1058.

Taub, E. (1976). Movement in nonhuman primates deprived of somatosensory feedback. *Exercise and Sport Science Review, 4*, 335–374.

Taub, E., Crago, J. E., Burgio, L. D., Groomes, T. E., Cook, E. W. III, DeLuca, S. C., et al. (1994). An operant approach to rehabilitation medicine: Overcoming learned nonuse by shaping. *Journal of the Experimental Analysis of Behavior, 61,* 281–293.

Taub, E., Miller, N. E., Novack, T. A., Cook, E. W. III, Fleming, W. C., Nepomuceno, C. S., et al. (1993). Technique to improve chronic motor deficit after stroke. *Archives of Physical Rehabilitation and Medicine, 74,* 347–354.

Taub, E., Uswatte, G., King, D. K., Morris, D., Crago, J. E., & Chatterjee, A. (2006). A placebo-controlled trial of constraint-induced movement therapy for upper extremity after stroke. *Stroke, 37,* 1045–1049.

Taub, E., Uswatte, G., & Pidikiti, R. (1999). Constraint-induced movement therapy: A new family of techniques with broad application to physical rehabilitation—A clinical review. *Journal of Rehabilitation Research and Development, 36,* 237–251.

Taylor, M. C., & Savin-Baden, M. (2001). Whose "evidence" are we applying? *British Journal of Occupational Therapy, 64,* 213.

Tham, K., & Tegnér, R. (1997). Video feedback in the rehabilitation of patients with unilateral neglect. *Archives of Physical Medicine and Rehabilitation, 78,* 410–413.

Thickbroom, G. W., Byrnes, M. L., Archer, S. A., & Mastaglia, F. L. (2004). Motor outcome after subcortical stroke correlates with the degree of cortical reorganization. *Clinical Neurophysiology, 115,* 2144–2150.

Thielman, G. T., Dean, C. M., & Gentile, A. M. (2004). Rehabilitation of reaching after stroke: Task-related training versus progressive resistive exercise. *Archives of Physical Medicine and Rehabilitation, 85,* 1613–1618.

Thomson, L. K. (1992). *Kohlman Evaluation of Living Skills* (3rd ed.). Bethesda, MD: American Occupational Therapy Association.

Tickle-Degnen, L. (1999). Organizing, evaluating, and using evidence in occupational therapy practice. *American Journal of Occupational Therapy, 53,* 537–539.

Tickle-Degnen, L. (2000). Evidence-based practice forum: Gathering current research evidence to enhance clinical reasoning. *American Journal of Occupational Therapy, 54,* 102–105.

Tickle-Degnen, L., Baker, N., & Murphy, S. (2001). The effectiveness of occupational therapy–related treatments for persons with Parkinson's disease: A meta-analysis review. *American Journal of Occupational Therapy, 55,* 385–392.

Tinetti, M. E. (1986). Performance-oriented assessment of mobility problems in elderly patients. *Journal of the American Geriatric Society, 34,* 119–126.

Toglia, J. P. (1993). *Contextual Memory Test (CMT).* Tucson, AZ: Therapy Skill Builders.

Toglia, J., & Kirk, U. (2000). Understanding awareness deficits following brain injury. *Neurorehabilitation, 15,* 57–70.

Trombly, C. A. (1995). Occupation: Purposefulness and meaningfulness as therapeutic mechanisms. *American Journal of Occupational Therapy, 49,* 960–972.

Trombly, C. A., & Ma, H.-I. (2002). A synthesis of the effects of occupational therapy on persons with stroke, part I: Restoration of roles, tasks, and activities. *American Journal of Occupational Therapy, 56,* 250–259.

Trombly, C. A., & Quintana, L. A. (1983). The effects of exercise on finger extension of CVA patients. *American Journal of Occupational Therapy, 37,* 195–202.

Trombly, C. A., Thayer-Nason, L., Bliss, G., Girard, C. A., Lyrist, L. A., & Brexa-Hooson, A. (1986). The effectiveness of therapy in improving finger extension in stroke patients. *American Journal of Occupational Therapy, 40,* 612–617.

Trombly, C. A., & Wu, C.-Y. (1999). Effect of rehabilitation tasks on organization of movement after stroke. *American Journal of Occupational Therapy, 53,* 333–344.

Turner-Stokes, L. (2003). Poststroke depression: Getting the full picture. *Lancet, 361,* 1757–1758.

Turton, A., & Fraser, C. (1990). The use of home therapy programmes for improving recovery of the upper limb following stroke. *British Journal of Occupational Therapy, 53,* 457–462.

Underwood, J., Clark, P. C., Blanton, S., Aycock, D. M., & Wolf, S. L. (2006). Pain, fatigue, and intensity of practice in people with stroke who are receiving constraint-induced movement therapy. *Physical Therapy, 86,* 1241–1250.

Uswatte, G., Taub, E., Morris, D., Barman, J., & Crago, J. (2006). Contribution of the shaping and restraint components of constraint-induced movement therapy to treatment outcome. *NeuroRehabilitation, 21,* 147–156.

van der Lee, J. H., Beckerman, H., Knol, D. L., de Vet, H. C. W., & Bouter, L. M. (2004). Clinimetric properties of the Motor Activity Log for the assessment of arm use in hemiparetic patients. *Stroke, 35,* 1410–1414.

van Heugten, C. M., Dekker, J., Deelman, B. G., Stehmann-Saris, J. C., & Kinebanian, A. (2000). Rehabilitation of stroke patients with apraxia: The role of additional cognitive and motor impairments. *Disability and Rehabilitation, 22,* 547–554.

van Heugten, C. M., Dekker, J., Deelman, B. G., van Dijk, A. J., Stehmann-Saris, J. C., & Kinebanian, A. (1998). Outcome of strategy training in stroke patients with apraxia: A phase II study. *Clinical Rehabilitation, 12,* 294–303.

Van Peppen, R. P., Kwakkel, G., Wood-Dauphinee, S., Hendriks, H. J., Van der Wees, P. J., & Dekker, J. (2004). The impact of physical therapy on functional outcomes after stroke: What's the evidence? *Clinical Rehabilitation, 18,* 833–862.

Vuagnat, H., & Chantraine, A. (2003). Shoulder pain in hemiplegia revisited: Contribution of functional electrical stimulation and other therapies. *Journal of Rehabilitation Medicine, 35,* 49–54.

Wade, D. T. (1992). Stroke: Rehabilitation and long-term care. *Lancet, 339,* 791–793.

Walker, M. F., Drummond, A. E. R., & Lincoln, N. B. (1996). Evaluation of dressing practice for stroke patients after discharge from hospital: A crossover design study. *Clinical Rehabilitation, 10,* 23–31.

Walker, M. F., Gladman, J. R., Lincoln, N. B., Siemonsma, P., & Whiteley, T. (1999). Occupational therapy for stroke patients not admitted to hospital: A randomised controlled trial. *Lancet, 354,* 278–280.

Walker, M. F., Leonardi-Bee, J., Bath, P., Langhorne, P., Dewey, M., Corr, S., et al. (2004). Individual patient data meta-analysis of randomized controlled trials of community occupational therapy for stroke patients. *Stroke, 35,* 2226–2232.

Wang, R. Y., Chen, H. I., Chen, C. Y., & Yang, Y. R. (2005). Efficacy of Bobath versus orthopaedic approach on impairment and function at different motor recovery stages after stroke. *Clinical Rehabilitation, 19,* 155–164.

Widen-Holmqvist, L., de Pedro-Cuesta, J., Holm, M., Sandstrom, B., Hellblom, A., Stawiarz, L., et al. (1993). Stroke rehabilitation in Stockholm: Basis for late intervention in patients living at home. *Scandinavian Journal of Rehabilitation Medicine, 25,* 173–181.

Wilson, D. J., Baker, L. L., & Craddock, J. A. (1984). Functional test for the hemiplegic upper extremity. *American Journal of Occupational Therapy, 38,* 159.

Winstein, C. J., & Knecht, H. G. (1990). Movement science and its relevance to physical therapy. *Physical Therapy, 70,* 759–762.

Winstein, C. J., Miller, J. P., Blanton, S., Taub, E., Uswatte, G., Morris, D., et al. (2003). Methods for a multisite randomized trial to investigate the effect of constraint-induced movement therapy in improving upper extremity function among adults recovering from a cerebrovascular stroke. *Neurorehabilitation and Neural Repair, 17,* 137–152.

Winstein, C. J., Rose, D. K., Tan, S. M., Lewthwaite, R., Chui, H. C., & Azen, S. P. (2004). A randomized controlled comparison of upper-extremity rehabilitation strategies in acute stroke: A pilot study of immediate and long-term outcomes. *Archives of Physical Medicine and Rehabilitation, 85*, 620–628.

Wittenberg, G. F., Chen, R., Ishii, K., Bushara, K. O., Eckloff, S., Croarkin, E., et al. (2003). Constraint-induced therapy in stroke: Magnetic-stimulation motor maps and cerebral activation. *Neurorehabilitation and Neural Repair, 17*, 48–57.

Woldag, H., & Hummelsheim, H. (2002). Evidence-based physiotherapeutic concepts for improving arm and hand function in stroke patients: A review. *Journal of Neurology, 249*, 518–528.

Wolf, S. L., Blanton, S., Baer, H., Breshears, J., & Butler, A. J. (2002). Repetitive task practice: A critical review of constraint-induced movement therapy in stroke. *Neurologist, 8*, 325–338.

Wolf, S. L., Catlin, P. A., Ellis, M., Link Archer, A., Morgan, B., & Piacentino, A. (2001). Assessing Wolf Motor Function Test as outcome measure for research inpatients after stroke. *Stroke, 32*, 1635–1639.

Wolf, S. L., Winstein, C. J., Miller, J. P., Taub, E., Uswatte, G., Morris, D., et al. (2006). Effect of constraint-induced movement therapy on upper extremity function 3 to 9 months after stroke: The EXCITE randomized clinical trial. *JAMA, 296*, 2095–2104.

Wolf, S. L., Winstein, C. J., Miller, J. P., Thompson, P. A., Taub, E., Uswatte, G., et al. (2008). Rentention of upper limb function in stroke survivors who have received constraint-induced movement therapy: The EXCITE randomized trial. *Lancet Neurology, 7*(1): 33–40.

Woodford, H., & Price, C. (2007). EMG biofeedback for the recovery of motor function after stroke. *Cochrane Database of Systematic Reviews*, Issue No. 2, Art. No. CD004585.

World Health Organization. (2001). *International classification of functioning, disability, and health.* Geneva, Switzerland: Author.

Wu, C.-Y., Chen, C. L., Tsai, W. C., Lin, K.-C., & Chou, S. H. (2007). A randomized controlled trial of modified constraint-induced movement therapy for elderly stroke survivors: Changes in motor impairment, daily functioning, and quality of life. *Archives of Physical Medicine and Rehabilitation, 88*, 273–278.

Wu, C.-Y., Lin, K.-C., Chen, H. C., Chen, I. H., & Hong, W. H. (2007). Effects of modified constraint-induced movement therapy on movement kinematics and daily function in patients with stroke: A kinematic study of motor control mechanisms. *Neurorehabilitation and Neural Repair, 21*, 460–466.

Wu, C., Trombly, C. A., Lin, K., & Tickle-Degnen, L. (1998). Effects of object affordances on reaching performance in persons with and without cerebrovascular accident. *American Journal of Occupational Therapy, 52*, 179–187.

Wu, C., Trombly, C. A., Lin, K., & Tickle-Degnen, L. (2000). A kinematic study of contextual effects on reaching performance in persons with and without stroke: Influences of object availability. *Archives of Physical Medicine and Rehabilitation, 81*, 95–101.

Young, G. C., Collins, D., & Hren, M. (1983). Effect of pairing scanning training with block design training in the remediation of perceptual problems in left hemiplegics. *Journal of Clinical Neuropsychology, 5*, 201–212.

Zinn, S., Dudley, T. K., Bosworth, H. B., Hoenig, H. M., Duncan, P. W., & Horner, R. D. (2004). The effect of poststroke cognitive impairment on rehabilitation process and functional outcome. *Archives of Physical Medicine and Rehabilitation, 85*, 1084–1090.

Zorowitz, R. D., Hughes, M. B., Idank, D., Ikai, T., & Johnston, M. V. (1996). Shoulder pain and subluxation after stroke: Correlation or coincidence? *American Journal of Occupational Therapy, 50*, 194–201.